EXPANDING HEALTH CARE HORIZONS

From a General Systems Concept of Health
To a National Health Policy

Second Edition

EXPANDING HEALTH CARE HORIZONS

From a General Systems Concept of Health
To a National Health Policy
Second Edition

HENRIK L. BLUM, M.D., M.P.H.

Professor
Department of Social and Administrative Health Services
School of Public Health
University of California, Berkeley

With a special Chapter 3

"EVIDENCE SUPPORTING A GENERAL SYSTEMS OR ECOLOGIC VIEW OF HEALTH"

Robert G. Robinson and **Henrik L. Blum**

Third Party Publishing Company
Oakland, California

EXPANDING HEALTH CARE HORIZONS: From a General Systems Concept of Health to a National Health Policy, Second Edition
Library of Congress Catalog Card Number: **82-084707**
International Standard Book Number: **0-89914-011-4**

Printed in the United States of America
First impression 1983
Third Party Publishing Company
A division of Third Party Associates, Inc.
P.O. Box 13306, Montclair Station
Oakland, California 94661

Design and editing by Paul R. Mico
Cover by Marilyn Amann

ACKNOWLEDGMENTS

I am very appreciative of the opportunity extended to me by Roslyn Lindheim, as coordinator, and Ivan Illich, as host and creator, of a seminar on "Health and Health Care," held in January, 1974 at CIDOC in Cuernevaca, Mexico to present rough outlines of many of these chapters. The extensive criticisms and clarifications which resulted have made this book more useful, I hope, but no less provocative. I am obligated to LuAnne Irion and Daniel Zwick for encouragement and to Jonathan Showstack for assistance in preparing the chapter on a National Health Policy, which appeared in the first edition, and to Christopher Bellavita for the many discussions which helped me prepare that chapter in this second edition.

I am also very indebted to my many students who, having perused these materials as part of their introduction to health and health care, offered many trenchant comments. I am likewise indebted to Robert Biller, Joseph Satten, Norman Sweet, Daniel Adelson, and Jonas Salk for various suggestions, key ideas, and words of support and warning, the latter not always heeded. Paul Mico and Neil Gilbert encouraged me, and Harry Specht did a tremendous job of editing the first edition which, although not always adhered to, did effect remarkable improvements in my estimation.

CONTENTS

LIST OF FIGURES

PROLOGUE

There is a presumption that health care and that portion of it known as medical care exist primarily for the purpose of improving health. Because there is reasonable doubt that this is really the case, there is ample reason to investigate this area of social implementation. In order to do so, the first step is to clarify the nature of health, how it is defined by social contexts, and what affects it. This is done in this book by means of applying the logic of general systems theory or of what may equally well be called an ecologic viewpoint. From an understanding of what produces good health and from a given viewpoint of what is socially desirable, it is then possible to deduce what is required of society in the way of institutions, relationships, services, and individual participation to improve health. This in turn calls for a National Health Policy which facilitates the achievement of what has been determined as necessary to improve health.

Society must also learn how to facilitate the meaningful updating of its definition of good health (what is desirable) as its needs and resources change. The changing social and physical environments that its members must face determine what capacities (health) and what health supports they must have if they are to thrive. Having the understanding of how its needs change, it is also to be hoped that society has the intelligence, will, and competence to redesign its values and goals as well as its National Health Policy and institutions for health or survival. Using these considerations as constraints, I suggest an approach to planning by means of which our society could proceed in the planning and creation of institutions which would promote well-being as we now define it, and at the same time continue to redefine it as needed. The policy proposal encompasses all of health care, but from time to time concentrates on medical care and its relationships with the emotional and social support services. All aspects of health promoting and maintaining services are seen as needing major reorientation, harnessing, and incorporation into a coherent National Health Policy, in order to bring about better health at costs that are bearable and in ways that offer suitable choices so that essentially all of us could find services acceptable to us.

Henrik L. Blum, M.D., M.P.H.
Berkeley, California
January, 1983

CHAPTER 1

FROM OUR UNDERSTANDINGS OF HEALTH, HEALTH CARE, AND MEDICAL CARE TO A NATIONAL HEALTH POLICY

There are three primary and wide-ranging concerns which prompted this text. The first is the **unsatisfactory state of our health** as compared to that which is presumably obtainable, already attained by many segments of our population, and by other nations. This is compounded by the inability of our increasingly expensive medical care activities to further improve health commensurate with its costs. The second is the **inequitable distribution of medical care services** so that large groups of people have great difficulty in reaching or entering the care delivery system to have their hurts, injuries, or health worries attended appropriately or in time. The third concern is for the unbelievably **rapid escalation of costs for medical care** which makes it harder for many to afford care. And because medical care takes an ever larger proportion of the Gross National Product, it becomes harder for the nation as a whole to find the financing necessary for other essential activities, such as rebuilding our dying urban centers, which has more to do with improving health than does medical care.

The first step in dealing with these concerns would appear to be a clarification of why satisfactory medical care cannot be equated with good health. But, to be more specific, we need to know what "health" is and what makes it "better" or "worse" before we suggest what "good health care" is, and what part of that task might be assigned to the providers of medical care and what part to others.

The title of this chapter suggests that we explain why health and medical care are more the concerns of social policy and social planning than of medicine or biologic science. It is therefore imperative to begin our inquiry with the question of how health is defined. In fact, each culture defines health according to its general belief systems. And what it wants in the way of health is part of its social policy and is an issue to be analyzed as part of its social planning.

At this point, a fuller comprehension of the factors that affect our well-being or health becomes critical. We must recurringly disentangle ourselves from current conventionally-wise or stereotyped belief-value systems about health if we are to acquire a clear picture of what is possible, what might wisely be wanted, and how we might achieve what is both possible and wanted. The relationship between medical care and health care, and of both to a national health policy, will become clearer as a consequence.

Three major streams of knowledge and theory have contributed to the creation of a systematic outlook on the origins of good and bad health. This book uses them as the basis for describing how to define and then promote health. All of these theories have not yet been widely accepted and thus they have not been employed as the means of guiding our social policies. However, they have the potential for unifying our understanding of a wide array of observations (accumulated by many disciplines and from all parts of the world), about which factors are associated with good and bad health. The reader will feel some relief to discover that many intuitions about health can now be given reasonable, even scientifically-elegant explanations.

One key stream of thought has been the development and application of a **general systems** or **ecologic view of the world** and of *homo sapiens*. The reader can trace this exciting development enjoyably through a few key works.[1] A second related stream of conceptualization is that of **feedback and cybernetic theory**.[2] The third critical stream is that of **observation, experimentation, and conceptualization about the manifestations of health.** It cannot be traced through any small list of writings, but several are landmarks.[3]

Once these three streams of thought are integrated into a comprehensible set of health paradigms, I find it possible to specify the nature and function of a "health or well-being promoting system," which is much more than a "medical care system." On analysis, these paradigms lead to stipulations about how a socially-concerned society can institutionalize mechanisms for sensitive perception and graceful change of posture required to make it into a socially conscious and wise society. My assumptions about such a society and my belief that it will care are, of course, major influences in directing this analysis.

The text utilizes the paradigms by drawing from them the parameters of a set of activities broadly defined as "well-being promotion and maintenance." Then, by way of example, it outlines one operational schema for comprehensive health and sickness services in a society which generally partakes of the mixed value configuration of present-day United States. It concludes with a description and brief analysis of a concordant National Health Policy which, I believe, would move the nation's efforts in the directions required to improve its health, to improve the equity of its distribution of health services, and to allow cost of such services to be kept at a desired level.

Politically, of course, the burning issues of medical care, such as frequent unavailability, unacceptability, inordinately-increasing expense, uneven quality, and iatrogenic (medically caused) damage must be faced now. Similarly, our obvious health deficiencies cannot be ignored. It is imperative, however, that we do not set about "correcting" problem after problem without a sense of where we want to be, or without guidance from our health paradigms as to how to get "there." Disjointed or blind incrementalism (patches) not only may eat up our resources but may detour us away from, or thwart the achievement of, our avowed major well-being goals.

A kind of combined short- and long-range planning is called for that requires a better understanding of the purposes of planning, where it can be done, and how it relates to policy setting. It also involves a better appreciation of how our value structure dictates what will and what will not be permitted. As a side issue, we learn that most planning tools are so value laden that, if used as their advocates suggest, the probable nature and shortcomings of their outcomes can generally be foreseen as soon as they are adopted for use in a given environment.[4]

Figure 1.1 makes the point that our culture lays out for us what are the acceptable views of "good" health (**Box A**) and thus sets the stage for the understanding of what can and should be done to maintain it and to correct its failures. Our culture likewise selects what roles the "good" society is to take in helping achieve "good" health of the individual and of the aggregate populace (**Box B**). These two value sets, in turn, determine those health and health care issues which members of a society will perceive as unbearable problems or as unattained goals (**Box C**). Similarly, the societal views of health and of its health services, as well as the perceived health-related issues will dictate the selection, education, and modes of practice of those who will be permitted to promote and restore health (**Box D**). **Box E** represents the subsequent deductions of the relevant professionals as to the nature of the needed institutions, skills, and processes that the "good" society will need and want in order to attain "good" health.

Box F represents our commonly accepted beliefs about why our people act the way they do. From this information we can postulate how we can harness motivations so as to create and utilize the needed institutions (**Box E**) appropriately. In **Box G**, we see the results of putting together all the prior information into a National Health Policy that lays out how we

FIGURE 1.1
GUIDANCE FROM A SOCIETY'S BELIEF AND VALUE SYSTEM:
THEY INSPIRE AND CONSTRAIN WHAT IS TAKEN INTO ACCOUNT IN DESIGNING
SUBSTANTIVE AND POLITICALLY-FEASIBLE INTERVENTIONS

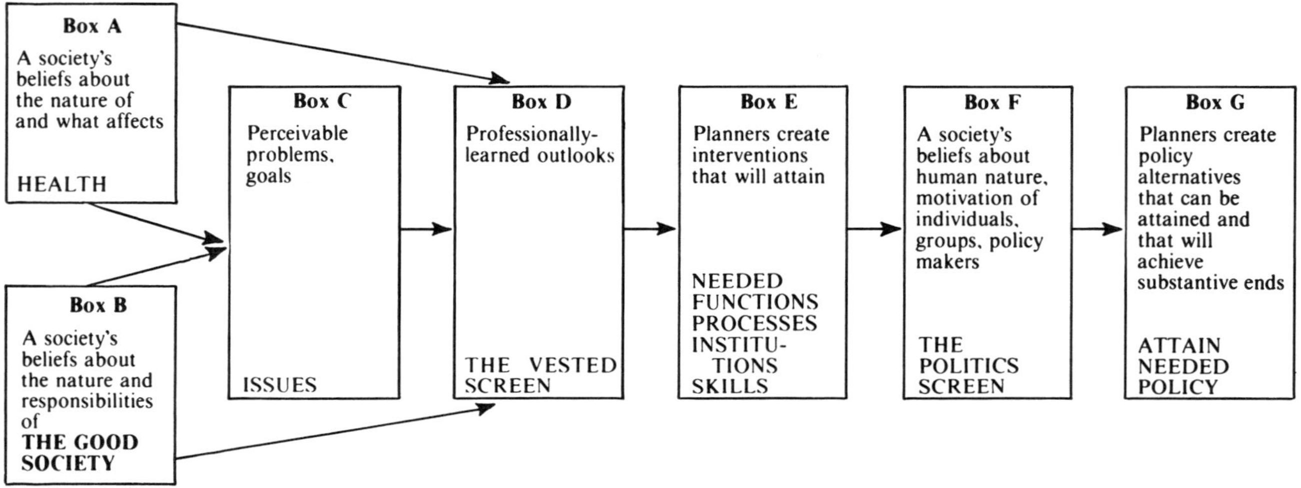

believe we can successfully finance, create, operate, and use the desired services (**Box E**) to resolve the perceived issues (**Box C**) and give us our "good" society and "good" health (**Boxes B** and **A**).

Sondra Koff describes this process well.[5] At the same time, we dare not overlook the fact that policies created for quite different purposes, such as for defense, conservation, foreign aid, education support, and so on, unintentionally may have major effects on our health.[6]

REFERENCES

1. L. von Bertalanffy, in A. Koestler and J. R. Smythies (Eds.), *Beyond Reductionism: New Perspectives in the Life Sciences,* New York: Macmillan, 1969. L. von Bertalanffy, "General Systems Theory," *General Systems,* 1956, 1, 1-10. H. Brody, "The Systems View of Man: Implications for Medicine, Sciences and Ethics," *Perspectives in Biology and Medicine,* 1973, 17:1 (Autumn), 71-92. A. Koestler, *Janus,* New York: Vintage, 1978, Appendix 1, 289-311. E. Laszlo, *The Systems View of The World,* New York: Braziller, 1972. J. G. Miller, "Living Systems: Basic Concepts," *Behavioral Sciences,* 1965, 10:3 (July), 193-237. A. Sheldon, In A. Sheldon, F. Baker, and C. P. McLaughlin (Eds.), *Systems and MedicalCare,* Cambridge, MIT Press, 1970, Chapter 5.

2. M. J. Apter, *Cybernetics and Development,* London, Pergamon, 1966. M. Maruyama, "The Second Cybernetics: Deviation Amplifying Mutual Casual Processes," In W. Buckley (ed.), *Modern Systems Researchfor the Behavioral Scientist,* Chicago, Aldine, 1968. N. Weiner, *Cybernetics,* Cambridge, MIT Press, 1948.

3. H. M. Brenner, "Fetal, Infant and Maternal Mortality During Periods of Economic Instability," *International Journal of Health Services,* 1973, 3:2, 145-159. R. Dubos, *Man Adapting,* New Haven, Yale University Press, 1965. G. L. Engel, "A Unified Concept of Health and Disease," *Perspectives in Biology and Medicine,* 1960, 3, 459-485. R. J. Haggerty, "The Boundaries of Health Care," *The Pharos,* AOA, 1972, (July) 106-111. L. Levi, *Society, Stress and Disease,* London, Oxford University Press, Vol. 1, 1971, Vol. 2, 1976. T. McKeown and C. R. Lowe, *An Introduction to Social Medicine,* Philadelphia, F. A. Davis Co., 1966, Chapter 1. J. Powles, "The Medicine of Industrial Man," *The Ecologist,* 1972, 2:10, 24-36. P. Sedgwick, "Illness—Mental and Otherwise," *The Hastings Center Studies,* 1973, 1:1, 19-40. H. E. Sigerist, *A History of Medicine,* New York, Oxford University Press, Vol. I, 1951, Vol. II, 1961. J. F. Fries and L. M. Crapow, *Vitality and Aging,* San Francisco, W. H. Freeman, 1981. T. McKeown, *The Role of Medicine,* New Jersey, Princeton University Press, 1979.

4. H. L. Blum *Planning For Health,* New York: Behavioral Publications, 2nd Edition, 1981, Chapters 5 and 7. D. B. Lee, Jr., "Requiem for Large Scale Models," *Journal of the American Institue of Planners,* 1973, 33:3, 163-178.

5. S. Z. Koff, "The Delivery of Health Care and Political Culture," *Policy Studies Journal,* 9:2, Special #1, 1980-81, 294-300.

6. N. Milio, *Promoting Health Through Public Policy,* Philadelphia, F. A. Davis, 1980.

Chapter 2

THE ECOLOGY OF HEALTH

I. *HOMO SAPIENS* AS A HIERARCHY OF NATURAL SYSTEMS: HEALTH AS A FUNCTION OF THE HARMONIOUSNESS OF INTER-RELATIONSHIPS BETWEEN SYSTEMS LEVELS

Poor health is seen as the outcome of forces which perturb or disrupt the harmonious interaction of the *homo sapiens* hierarchy of natural systems to the point where one or more system levels are malfunctioning (**Figure 2.1**).[1] This may not be beyond the point where recuperation and even strengthening of the system may result. Examples of the latter are as omnipresent and diverse as the immune mechanisms set in motion by infections or the capacity to increasingly cope with reoccurrences of stressful demands which initially were debilitating events. The idea of increasing strength as a result of surviving and building resistance has, in some quarters, come to be known as *General Adaptation Theory* and in others as *Morphogenesis.*

The basic concepts of general systems theory which we use in this essay are presented in this chapter. General systems theory allows us to view *homo sapiens* in a particularly dynamic way and health as a consequence of a predictable but immensely diverse set of forces.

Laszlo's description of **four attributes of natural systems** offers a useful starting point.[2]

A. One: Natural Systems are Wholes With Irreductible Properties

Each system is more than the sum of its parts. Its formal structure is built up out of its parts and partakes of the characteristic interdependent

FIGURE 2.1
THE HOMO SAPIENS HIERARCHY OF NATURAL SYSTEMS AND THE NATURE OF FEEDBACK MECHAMISMS

Person level	System level	Means of feedback
p+6	biosphere	
		use of resources and deposition of wastes (environ cycles)
p+5	homo sapiens	
		life styles, behaviors derived and symbolized from values and norms set by successful species responses to environment
p+4	cultures	
		economic and political forces
p+3	nations (societies)	
		exchange of policies, symbols, goods, resources
p+2	communities and organizations	
		exchange of policies, symbols, goods, resources
p+1	families	
		interpersonal and symbolic communications
p	persons: social, psychic, somatic	intrapersonal resolution of memory conditioning, learning, imagining, desiring, valuing, interacting with the interpersonal and physiologic realms
		physiologic and sensory awareness
p-1	body systems	
		neural impulses, hormones
p-2	organs	
		ionic equilibria, fluid flow, permeability, active transport
p-3	tissues	
		ionic equilibria, fluid flow, permeability, active transport
p-4	cells	
		enzymes, gene activators and repressors, ionic equilibria
p-5	molecules	
		chemical bonds, reactions, electrostatic forces
p-6	atoms	
		electrostatic forces
p-7	subatomic particles	

Adapted from H. Brody "The Systems View of Man: Implications for Medicine, Science and Ethics," *Perspectives in Biology and Medicine*, Autumn 1973, 71-91.

relationships of these parts. Parts generally cannot be removed without altering the wholeness, oneness, nature, function, and often the viability of the system.

Whether the natural system is an atom built up out of its lesser parts, the liver built up out of its tissues, or a family of persons composed of its members, the system is a distinctive whole made up of interrelating and interdependent parts that give it its unique characteristics.

Similarly, each of the other three million species contained in and making up the biosphere has a distinctive hierarchy of natural systems, each of which has its distinctive parts, forms, and relationships. To clarify our meaning, **species** is a term used to designate the most inclusive group of individuals that has the potential for interbreeding and production of fertile offspring. Thus, all humans are included in the species *homo sapiens.*[3]

Laszlo states that evolution has super-imposed encompassing system upon system in a continuous hierarchy (see **Figure 2.1**). These range from the simplest or sub-organic systems (which is the subject matter of the physical sciences), to and through the range of organic and living systems (which is the subject matter of the biologic sciences), to and through the realm of the supra-organic systems (which is the subject matter of the social sciences). At the level of the biosphere, all the sciences are called into play. Laszlo also points out that systems that are hierarchically organized are the only ones likely to survive because hierarchical systems can be decomposed to their various levels of subsystems without thereby ruining their entire organization. On the other hand, when nonhierarchic systems are disbalanced, they come completely unstuck, disaggregating to their elementary constituents.

B. Two: Natural Systems Maintain Themselves in a Changing Environment

In contrast to physical objects, such as houses or cars, which inevitably wear out even with the best of care, natural systems are self-repairing and self-maintaining by means of energy taken in from one or another level of the systems above or below it in the hierarchy. The ongoing acquisition and use of energy, the creation of material or energy, and the disposal of wastes is what typifies a natural system as an **open system in a steady state**. The **person** is such a system: so are his or her sub-systems, such as the brain, or a red blood cell, or a sodium atom; and so are the supra-systems such as the family or nation.

Any system has somewhat predictable limits of survival, and aging and death are normal and necessary phases. With aging, the system's self-replenishment goes on less and less effectively, but its death may come slowly or rapidly. The life span of a system in the *homo sapiens* hierarchy may range from a fraction of a second for some molecules, a hundred years for persons, thousands of years for cultures, to billions of years for our biosphere-containing planet.

Most living systems are able to maintain themselves by means of reproduction which, however, is not always effected. The capacity to replace and replenish is a necessary precondition for life.

Social or supra-organic systems, like living organisms, continuously attempt to maintain homeostasis or an optimal equilibrium. But they typically have more leeway and there are more vigorously changing relationships of the parts to the whole and to one another. These result in a shifting of equilibrium and emergence of new social systems. Sometimes, "offsprings" are indeed extruded, at other times death of the system occurs, at others there is reformulation of any remaining sub-systems into new supra-systems.

Homeostasis or **equilibrium** carries the connotation that systems are able to resist or overcome forces which threaten disruption to their optimally relating and functioning internal elements within widely varying limits. Calling upon extra capacities which it directly commands in the form of support from supra-systems and sub-systems, a system, by means of its feedback loop communications, generally copes with the day-to-day forces imposed on it and returns to its optimal state of equilibrium or homeostasis. Even after a particularly rigorous upsetting thrust, the system may return to an apparently completely normal capacity and life expectancy. Typically, as has already been noted, it learns how to carry such thrusts and may emerge stronger in respect to comparable perturbations which it confronts in the future.

At other times, a system returns to apparently normal function but with lessened reserve. As a result, it may have future episodes of failing and a shortened life expectancy as well. Sometimes, adequate equilibrium can be maintained only by artificial substitution of function or substances, or by use of interventions which counteract the force that is upsetting the equilibrium. It may be necessary to counteract the activities of supra- or sub-systems that customarily put demands on the ailing system or to support them in activities now running at dangerous levels as a result of the ailing system. In some situations, disturbing forces are predictable, and they can be kept from forming or be kept isolated, or the at-risk system can be strengthened in advance to cope with them.

Most excitingly, systems may innovate as by mutation, or they may join forces with others, or create new systems able to avoid, destroy or override feared perturbations. A system's equilibrium may slowly be shifted, as when chronic malnutrition results in smaller people able to survive on fewer calories. Unfortunately, this probably represents a sub-optimal equilibration. At a higher systems level, endless aggression may drive persons to exist in fortified cities. This may be generally advantageous or disadvantageous as it leads to formation of new kinds of social systems.

C. Three: Natural Systems Create Themselves in Response to the Challenge of the Environment

Homeostasis and equilibrium are not the only ways in which natural systems maintain themselves in a changing environment. The lowest or sub-organic systems in the *homo sapiens* hierarchy are the most homeostatic and restricted to maintain structure within established limits. But as we ascend into the organic systems and on up to the person and higher levels, we accept guidance from Buckley[4] and Koestler[5] and note that the higher systems are regarded as **complex adaptive systems** because they are in constant change (even though at any one moment they may be perceived as attempting to maintain homeostasis) as a result of their responses to feedback or lack thereof from other systems. The concept of seeking or at least utilizing change, rather than battling for homeostasis at the sub-organic and person levels, is generally spoken of as growth or maturation.

At higher-systems levels, the ability to shift structure and function in adapting to changing circumstances has also been called **morphogenesis.**[6] And whether we think of systems, such as families, or those as high up as societies, we have the imagery of clinging to the old but needing and accepting the new.

Thus we come to the third rule, **Natural Systems Create Themselves in Response to the Challenge of the Environment**. When we comprehend this duality of homeostasis and morphogenesis, it commences to matter little whether a system which has changed under our observation essentially has died and been replaced or has metamorphosed.

Self-creation is a typical system response to changing conditions or to an environment whose nature or forces are such that the system, as it is constituted, cannot satisfactorily cope with such forces by less than changes in its existing structure, i.e., becoming a new system. This is a precondition for evolution which represents the successful replacement of one system by another, and, subsequently, often of one species by another that can cope better with the current conditions. Natural systems evolve new structures and new functions over time, whether it be as a result of cellular-level mutations or changes in value and behavior patterns in societies. Notwithstanding, even the highest natural systems often cannot cope with rapid or major environmental changes; the evidence is all around us that many species and societies have perished and are known to us only as entombed remains.

Laszlo reminds us that creation of new or altered systems is the evolutionary process of phylogenesis which, in spite of some interesting resemblances, is not the same as natural maturation or predetermined ontogenesis, i.e., the processes that an organism passes through from birth to death. The latter are also true changes in a system arising as a result of changes in interaction and feedback with and among its sub-systems; they are precoded genetically, from which there can be no deviation. Phylogenesis, however, is the result of open interaction among systems as they respond to changes in one another, for each is part of the environment of the others. A system that "invents" a new attribute or behavior does so randomly. Although such mutations are generally associated with less capacity for survival, an occasional one provides the system with more adaptive capacity and, thus, may come to replace the systems from which it arose. Sometimes, the nature of the invention is in relating to or living closely with other systems, as in the formation of nations, super organizations, commune families, or commensal and symbiotic relationships. Where one of the two joiners hurts the other, the relationship is parasitic and is usually shortened in accordance with the degree of the hurt.

D. Four: Natural Systems are Coordinating Interfaces in Nature's Hierarchies

In a given species hierarchy of systems, each level of system links those immediately below with the one directly above. The number of systems at the bottom of the hierarchy are myriad, and there is a continuous decline in the number of systems as we go up the pyramid of systems to the level of the single biosphere. Each system is a whole in respect to its parts, and the parts are wholes with respect to one another and with the next higher level whole.

An individual system forms the coordinating interfaces for its supra-system, its many sub-systems, and with its environment. Influences transmitted from within a sub-system are easily visualized at the sub-organic level of molecules, atoms, and sub-atomic particles. At the organic level, the cells integrate their sub-cellular entities and relate to tissues, the tissues organize their cells and relate to organs, and so on. However, it should not be assumed that these interfaces are necessarily tidy or concise boundaries. They may be more like loose nets, or extended and intricately devolved pipe-like systems, as easily witnessed in some of the immunity or guarding tissues and the blood or lymph systems.

At the supra-organic level in the *homo sapiens* hierarchy, the same kind of interrelationships are observable in the role of the parents (family) in socializing the child. However, at the supra-organic levels, where the person is so highly integrated with his or her sub-systems, yet so freely mobile in regard to the supra-systems, the interfaces are particularly diffuse. The person contains unusual perceptive, reasoning, imagining, and inventing attributes, as well as a prodigious memory, memory aids, and mechanical repositories of beliefs and values. As a result, the person's supra-systems have invented innumerable supra-organic (i.e., social) systems that relate him or her horizontally and vertically in many ways not indicated by the schematic *homo sapiens* hierarchy described in **Figure 2.1**. These auxiliary nets (which might be considered as alternative ways of conceptualizing the supra-organic levels of systems) include political, administrative, judicial, economic, professional, and employment patterns of relationships. As a consequence, the system interfaces at the *homo sapiens* supra-organic level are particularly diffuse, complex, and extended. Some readers of this material have suggested, for this reason, that a better term for the *homo sapiens* "hierarchy of systems" would be "an increasingly encompassing set of nets."

Feedback, the means of controlling, influencing, or communicating between a system, its supra-system, or its sub-systems takes many forms. Feedback involves a mutual cause-effect relationship. In sub-organic or physical systems, feedback involves force potentials; in organic or living systems, they are more often physio-chemical means. In supra-systems, as between persons or organizations of persons, they take the form of communications, such as signals, symbols, speech, writings, exchange of policies, symbols and goods, and interpersonal behavior. When we discuss environments in the general systems sense, the great environ cycles of energy, carbon, water, and so on will be seen as still another kind of nutrient-moving feedback which relates everything under the biosphere, as well as the geo-chemical resources of the planet and energy of the sun. To provide the quickest review of the nature of feedback mechanisms, **Figure 2.1** is presented as adapted from Brody.[8]

Not all feedback goes directly from one system level to another. Some communications leap-frog one or many systems levels; some influence many systems levels of a hierarchy simultaneously.

By virtue of its means of influencing and being influenced, each system acts as a whole and in its own right, no matter how many or complex its levels of sub- and supra-systems. At the person-system level, the feedback loops connect the person to his or her sub-systems by mostly neuro-electric-physio-chemical mechanisms. However, the person also responds to a comparison of one's perceptions, beliefs, imagination, and desires as to how one should be and how one feels him- or herself to be. Affective and intellectual stimuli, as well as sensory capacities, advise one how others perceive him or her. A significant example is the patient who assumes he is critically ill because of how he interprets his doctor's reactions; another is the "primitive" who dies because he perceives he has been bewitched.

These varied mechanisms make feedback a particularly complicated phenomenon. In fact, when we accommodate to the well-verified observations that such physiologic entities as blood pressure, oxygen consumption, and heart rate can be altered by subjective concentration, we get an idea of how tangible, pervasive, and interrelated are the communicating or mutually-controlling feedback mechanisms.[9] The long history of Yoga attests to the sophisticated levels at which mind-body feedback technology has been understood and utilized.

Some feedback mechanisms, the so-called negative ones, normally act so as to activate mechanisms which return the system it serves to its prior or customary state and, thus, attempt to maintain homeostasis (e.g., acid-base balance as manifested by the pH of the blood). Others, the so-called positive ones, act so as to report deviation and encourage mechanisms which increase deviation of the same kind. These are not uncommon. Examples are the inexorable maturation process of the individual from one state of development to the next, and the extension of profitable economic or political conquest processes of one nation over another.

E. The Environment in Systems Terms

In the earlier description of the *homo sapiens* hierarchy of systems, the biosphere was arbitrarily designated as the highest level of system to be considered in our discussion. The biosphere is a narrow envelope of air, water, and soil at the periphery of the earth. It extends approximately seven miles above and seven miles below sea level. In it are to be found all living species.

By portraying the biosphere as the most encompassing, or highest, system of concern in the *homo sapiens* hierarchy, we do not mean to imply that it is the captive or property of the species *homo sapiens*. It equally includes another three million living species hierarchies, each of which equally claims the biosphere as the top or most encompassing system in its hierarchy. Each one of those three million system hierarchies is part of the environment for the others. The human-kind hierarchical set of systems is potentially juxtaposed at every one of its levels to each and any level of each of the other three million species hierarchies.

Just as the biosphere is the "top" supra-system of our earth, and all of its sub-systems are the environment for all the species, each system level in a given species hierarchy is likewise the master supra-system for all systems beneath it. The next most encompassing system in the *homo sapiens* hierarchy is, therefore, that of *homo sapiens*. The human species can be sub-divided into innumerable cultures, each of which is further subdivisible into nations (societies), and so on. What, then, is the environment of one person in the systems view? It consists immediately of the other individual members of the family, and of the family as a unit *per se*, for it is the person's next higher controlling system. One's environment also consists of community and various organizations, all the families contained therein, and all their members. It also consists of one's nation and of all the communities, organizations, families, and individuals so embraced. It also consists of one's culture and all the nations sharing it, with their communities, organizations, families, and individual persons. And so on, up to the biosphere and all of its three million species hierarchies and of the individuals within them.

What we have portrayed is the person's environment on the grand scale. However, in order to describe the effects of environment on a person's health, we must be more specific and definitive about his or her environment. Here, the concept of **ecosystem** is useful.

Ecoystems To clarify the nature of a person's "working" environment, it is helpful to delineate systems in another way. We can regard the biosphere as the master earth-based ecosystem, in which gaseous, aqueous, and mineral entities interact with one another and with all living species. An **ecoystem**, by definition, includes all the living species to be found in an area defined by some meaningful but arbitrarily-limited set of boundaries. It also includes their reactions with one another and with the inanimate materials that affect their lives in any significant way. The biosphere, the largest of the ecosystems which we shall consider, is neatly bounded.

The concept of ecosystems allows us to subdivide the biosphere not only by species hierarchies, but also into smaller subdivisions of ecosystems and hierarchies of ecosystems. These may be spatially designated areas, such as the sky, a sea, continent, forest, plain, desert, lake, and so on. All of the species and minerals that act or react in the named ecosystem territory are part of that ecosystem. Such large ecosystems, in turn, can be subdivided into smaller ones that help one understand certain kinds of actions and reactions taking place in that area. Thus, for some purposes, the seashore is an ideal ecosystem, and so is an alfalfa field or a rotting log. The *homo sapiens* hierarchy or any of its sub-systems, including human artifactual productions, such as machines or the plants and animals that *homo sapiens* breeds and raises, may be present in any given ecosystem. And when they are, they become part of that ecosystem. Directly or indirectly, individuals and groups from the *homo sapiens* hierarchy have made themselves critical ingredients of most significant ecosystems.

Ecosystems are described not only by their arbitrarily-chosen boundaries but by the rates of circulation of any species or minerals within those boundaries, and by the rates of flows of individuals, energy, and matter across its boundaries.[10] In an ongoing or stable ecosystem, its elements are specific and separate, yet intrinsically interrelated. Each species supports the others directly and indirectly.

Environ Cycles Focusing on the ecosystem, whether it be a continent or a tide pool, brings out the specific relationships of the living and of the inanimate. The concept of **environ cycle** is a useful way to illustrate these relationships, in order to understand how the ecosystem maintains itself. We all know of specific behaviors that have upset certain ecologic balances. An example is the excessive nitrogenation of food-producing fields which grossly disturbs life in the waters receiving the abnormally nitrogen-rich run-offs. Similarly, we have observed how the use of herbicides and pesticides may spill out of a particular ecosystem, and even contaminate the entire biosphere with effects that threaten so many species that *homo sapiens* is itself threatened. These are special cycles that are swept up into the major environ cycles and must be understood if man is to guide behavior appropriately.

Environ cycles are the bio-geo-chemical nets, flows, and exchanges that interrelate the sub-organic (or mineral) system, the living (or organic) ones, and the social (or supra-organic) ones. The major cycles, such as those of energy, water, carbon, nitrogen, and phosphorous, are interrelating webs that can be conceived of as the feedback or communication loops that guide and mediate the survival, distribution, perturbations, evolution, and disappearance of any of the hierarchical species systems or of their sub-systems.

The major environ cycles are affected by, and affect most of, our undertakings. Some environ cycles are built on vast and accessible reserves and are carried on by complex and redundant pathways, so that the societies of *homo sapiens* have difficulty in upsetting them. Other environ cycles are cycling more precariously with limited reserves and, as they lose their resources or *modus operandi*, the inhabitants of the ecosystems dependent on them will suffer accordingly.

Let us consider one environ cycle or feedback loop that unites all ecosystems and all species hierarchies of systems. The **world nitrogen cycle** is one of the most instructive, as well as critical, to the survival of living systems.[11] Its functioning illustrates how inorganic resources are moved about by natural organic or living and inorganic geo-chemical activities, as well as by the social forces, knowledge, and behavior of *homo sapiens* which represent the uses and abuses of nitrogen. These uses, combined with frequently unwise distribution policies for resources, result in truly frightening population effects. This cycle interrelates with the energy cycle, as *homo sapiens* acts to fix or obtain and move nitrogen and to move the water required to take advantage of the plant growth made possible by increased nitrogen supplies.

The capacity of *homo sapiens* to change supra-organic systems, as well as to alter other species hierarchies, is further exemplified by the ability to alter genetic constructs of other matter-creating species in order to increase food supplies. The green revolution seems to have made countries, such as India, potentially or actually self-sufficient in meeting their calorie needs.[12] However, an unchanged social outlook, reinforced by differential economic, educational, and cultural capacities to carry off agricultural change, will probably lead the green revolution to larger scale, privately-owned farming with heavy equipment. This will displace former agricultural workers who, in an under-employed, poverty-stricken society, have neither skills nor opportunities to do anything else. Nor can they buy the increased food production for there has been no distribution of the gains of the country's increased production. Worker wages may, in fact, decline. Thus, India's green revolution may result in an increasing proportion of the population suffering from starvation.[13]

To further complicate matters, non-renewable energy reserves presently provide the increased energy needed to obtain the water and fertilizer required for the green revolution to be successful. This energy is not always available, and when it is its costs may increase drastically. As food prices subsequently go up, starvation will extend. Where individual growers garner riches, often by exporting the food their own people need, their new earnings typically bring back relatively-useless luxury goods or heavy equipment to replace more workers and use more fuel. It is ironic, too, that large-tract modern agriculture may also mean less production of protein-rich legumes.[14] Moreover, the new grains typically have much less protein than the older strains of wheat, corn, or rice that they replace. It is true that good protein is destroyed to produce human energy if there is an inadequate calorie intake, but for lack of distributive justice, as well as a lower proportionate availability of protein, the new look may find more people with less calories and less protein as well.

The newly-engineered genetic constructs that may give us better protein and require less or no additional nitrogen or water may minimize or worsen the stranglehold of the well-to-do over the survival of the less-well-off in differing situations. Further debated complications, such as increased weeds and needs for herbicides, need for more pesticides to protect genetically less disease-resistant mass plantings, increased fertilizer run-offs that poison streams and larger bodies of water, and massive erosion or soil quality deterioration, suggest that all is far from well with man's greatest interventive "triumphs" in agriculture.[15]

We see how political and social beliefs and institutions of *homo sapiens* dictate the manipulation of the environ cycles and alter the well-being and survivability of large groups of *homo sapiens*, as well as of innumerable other species. There are many sources of information about human attempts at interventions, their potentialities, and their outcomes.[16]

F. Spread of Perturbations: A Key Attribute of a Species Hierarchy of Systems

From what has been said about the attributes of systems, it is apparent that systems occur in hierarchies. Brody has described such a hierarchy for the species *homo sapiens* (**Figure 2.1**).[17] A few major generalizations can now be made about the relationships of one system level to another, inside such a hierarchy.

Perturbations in one system level may spread to others The application of a force at the level of any system will tax the homcostatic mechanisms of that system to buffer or overcome that force. Because a system (**s**) interfaces, and is an interactant with the system directly above it (**s+1**) and the one directly below it (**s–1**), much of its homeostatic capacities are directly obtained from them, particularly from the sub-systems.

Some forces overcome the homeostatic mechanisms of the system affected initially (**s**), and this disordered system in turn becomes a disrupting force on the system directly above it (**s+1**) and the one directly below it (**s–1**). The more it is disturbed or damaged, the less it is able to coordinate and interrelate its own sub-systems, and the more they will fall into chaotic and destructive interplay. A sub-system (**s–1**), thus injured, passes on its disrupting status to its own sub-systems (**s–2**) as well as back to its immediate supra-system (**s**), which was the site of the initial force and failure and which is now further deranged.

Similarly, the more the initially affected system (**s**) is disequilibrized, the more likely it is to disrupt the system above it, of which it is a necessary and distinguishing component. If the supra-system (**s+1**) is unable to contain the thrust of the failing system (**s**), it will in turn become a disorganizing force for its supra-system (**s+2**) and at the same time a further destructive force for its sub-system (**s**), which was the initial seat of failure.

Thus, the waves of perturbation or disequilibration may spread upward and downward from the system affected by the initial untoward force.

Because we generally focus on the well-being of individuals, the individual person is the system we are going to place at the center of our discussion. Brody (**Figure 2.1**) has visualized a hierarchy of systems for *homo sapiens* which puts the person-level of system at the center. We can label the person as **p** and the hierarchy of systems above as **p+1** through **p+6**, and those below as **p–1** to **p–7**. We can then describe the flow of perturbations up and down the *homo sapiens* systems hierarchy, and can visualize how the well-being of a person is both a consequence of, and a factor in, producing the flow of perturbations.

Perturbations spreading from higher to lower systems are likely to produce extensive and diverse effects Because the supra-systems are, or

FIGURE 2.2
DOWNWARD SPREAD OF PERTURBATIONS

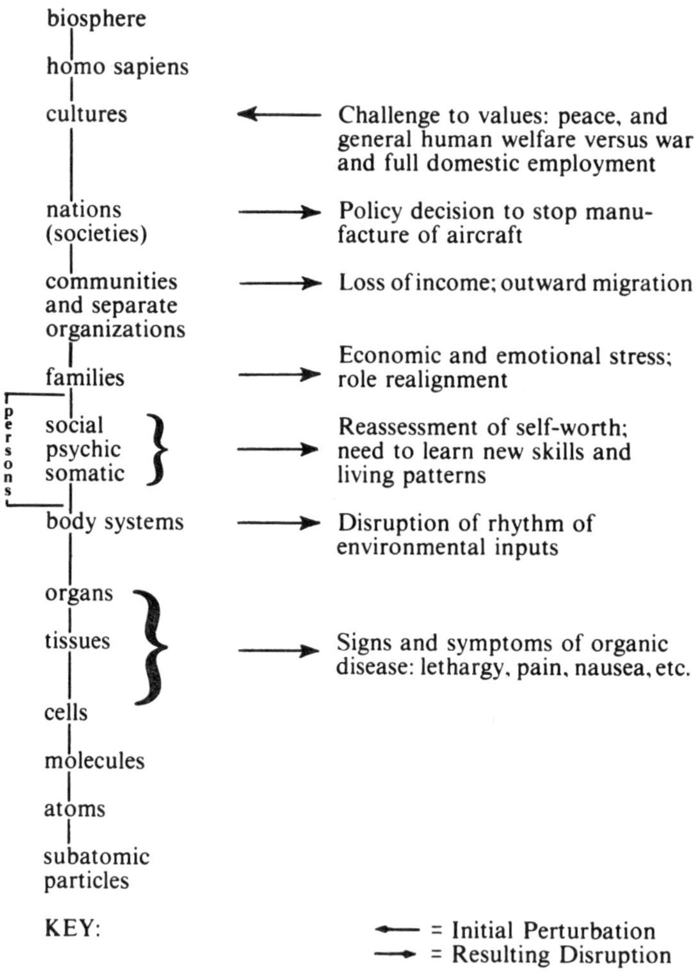

(Disease example. Stress-related psychosomatic illness in a post-Vietnam unemployed aerospace engineer: example of spread of disruption downward through the hierarchy).

Adapted from H. Brody "The Systems View of Man: Implications for Medicine, Science and Ethics," *Perspectives in Biology and Medicine*, Autumn 1973, 71-91.

control, the environment for their lower or sub-systems, it is easy to see how the disruption of a higher-level system spreads out and may involve all lower systems (**Figure 2.2**).

Perturbations also spread from lower systems to higher ones Because persons are dependent on their sub-systems, and supra-organic systems are dependent on persons, it is easy to visualize how failures or perturbations can spread upward (**Figure 2.3**).

In the case of species-fixed or genetically-encoded life spans, organic-level systems begin to fail as scheduled. It is clear that disturbed lower-level systems thereby put stress on the person-level, and disturbances there put stress on higher-level systems. Where individual persons, such as Woodrow Wilson or Joseph Stalin, have become key or controlling in the supra-organic systems, history helps us visualize how their somatic, psychic, or social illnesses affect the destiny and well-being not only of their families but of many and, occasionally, of most peoples of the world.

Perturbations act circularly A perturbation starting in a higher-system comes to affect various lower-systems, whose resultant perturbations may then go on to upset the initiating or other higher-level systems. Disruption in a system can obviously also spread up and down at the same time.

Perturbation is illness A perturbed system is one that is out of equilibrium, and perturbation is another way of saying ill-health.

II. HEALTH: THE QUALITY OF FUNCTIONING OF THE PERSON-LEVEL SYSTEM

The smooth functioning of the person-level system is good health. The health status of the individual person is determined by the degree of harmonious interaction among the various system levels in the *homo sapiens* hierarchy.[18] The causes of ill-health are not, therefore, free-standing intrusive or deprivatory episodes thrust upon a given individual. They arise from disturbed relationships in a system, or between systems levels, as one or another system is driven to malfunctioning by forces from above (external) or below (internal) that overcome its own homeostatic capacities to muffle or absorb perturbations, or that exceed the support capacity of its own superior and inferior systems.

FIGURE 2.3
UPWARD SPREAD OF PERTURBATIONS

biosphere	⟶	Resource drain
homo sapiens	⟶	Loss of individual from gene pool (self-adjusting)
cultures	⟶	Challenge to traditional values: desire to care for sick vs. competing uses for resources
nations (societies)	⟶	Challenge to resource-allocation and welfare policies
communities and organizations	⟶	Resources diverted for care of sick individual
families	⟶	Emotional trauma, distorted relationships, economic drain
person: social, psychic, somatic	⟶	Inability to perform complex, coordinated physical and mental activities
body systems, organs, tissues	⟶	Arrested development
cells	⟶	Mutant gene on chromosome Lack of directions for differentiation
molecules	⟶	Alteration of DNA template
atoms	⟶	Electron excitation and escape
subatomic particles	⟵	Photons of radiation (upon gamete)

KEY:

⟵ = Initial perturbation
⟶ = Resulting Disruption

(Disease example. Severe physical and mental retardation caused by a radiation-induced mutation in the gamete: example of spread of disruption upward through the hierarchy).

Adapted from H. Brody "The Systems View of Man: Implications for Medicine, Science and Ethics," *Perspectives in Biology and Medicine*, Autumn 1973, 71-91.

A. A Description of Health

In **Figure 2.4**, we consider 12 distinctive facets of the somatic, psychic, and social aspects of health that encompass a relatively-full meaning of health in our society. The 12 facets are presented in terms of either **positive** (good health) or **negative** (bad health), in accordance with customary usages. From a systems viewpoint of the determinants of health, it seems wise to consider all departures from good health as negatively-regarded deviances from social expectations, rather than as "true" abnormalities.[19]

The brief descriptions of each of the 12 facets of health suggest, and documentation supports, the belief that there are reasonable means of identifying and measuring each of the facets.[20]

Placing these 12 facets or criteria of health side-by-side poses problems for some observers, because on first glance they appear to have quite different properties. However, they are built up as suitable indicators of functionality and adaptivity (or dysfunctionality and maladaptivity) of the person-level of system. The person's well-being as a whole system cannot be defined by anything less than a review of one's overall systemic functioning. No matter how that functioning is subdivided and defined by society, it has interrelated and indivisible social, psychic, and somatic components as the person-system interfaces with its supra- and sub-systems.

From the general systems point of view, it is useful to describe the health of the person as the composite of three interacting and hierarchically-related person-level areas: the **somatic** (i.e., product of the person's internal or organic and sub-organic system levels), the **psychic** (i.e., integrating function), and the **social** (i.e., supra-system interactant level).

Of course, the somatic, psychic, and social integrating levels cannot be separated. The person is a physiologically-integrated and structured whole, composed of sub-systems. One receives (or feels) messages from the sub-systems which tell one of external and internal, and of normal or abnormal, pressures and states of affairs bearing upon the person. At the same time, one is a sociologically-integrated or directed sub-system observing and feeling the influences of the supra-organic levels of the *homo sapiens* hierarchy. Because one interfaces or connects these two streams, he or she is most distinctively a feeling, psychological, thinking, and reflective entity as well.

Much of what one knows, believes, and is able to imagine stems from participation in the supra-organic systems. Yet psychologic feedback, in part, determines what one's inputs will be into the supra-organic systems. The capacity to receive, to be guided by, and to react to each set of messages from above and below is distinctively and psychologically "him" or "her." The ability to indulge in self-reflection, as well as to perceive and react, further modifies one's receptivity and behavior. It is an exquisitely-

FIGURE 2.4
TWELVE MEASURABLE ASPECTS OF THE STATE OF HEALTH

Life expectancy or duration The length of survival is usually expressed as the average years of survival for a selected group or as the degree of prematurity of death as compared to some selected standards (a somatic descriptor).

Impairment (Disease or Infirmity) Departure from accepted physiologic, psychologic, or anatomic structural norms appropriate to age and sex (a somatic or psychic decriptor).

Discomfort or illness Feelings of distress in a person (may be a somatic, psychic, or social descriptor, and is generally a combination).

Disability or incapacity Inability of a person to fully carry out customary or expected duties for his or her age, sex, and social roles in his or her society whether due to functional incapacity or social labeling. It is to be noted that **handicapping is defined as a disadvantage for an individual resulting from an impairment or a disability** (may be a somatic, psychic, or social descriptor, and is generally a combination).

Participation in health care Capacity or willingness to share with health service providers in the work of keeping oneself healthy or returning to better health (primarily a descriptor of social health, although often dependent on somatic and psychic interactants).

Health behavior Acts, or style of life, which directly support or threaten health. This includes such behavior as smoking, drinking, risky driving, irregular rest, and so on (a social descriptor primarily).

Ecologic behavior A person's willed or reflex acts and attitudes towards other species, natural resources, and ecosystems (a social descriptor).

Social behavior A person's willed or reflex acts and attitudes towards others of his or her species at the person, family, community, and organization or national level, such as willingness to help, rob, despoil, or murder (a social descriptor which may have large psychic elements).

Interpersonal relationships Quality of communications with others (essentially a psychic descriptor, but one that is heavily affected by somatic and social health).

Reserve or positive health Resistance to disease or the capacity to endure unusual somatic, psychic, or social pressures, (a combination descriptor of somatic, psychic, and social interactants).

FIGURE 2.4
TWELVE MEASURABLE ASPECTS OF
THE STATE OF HEALTH, continued

External satisfaction Sense of enjoyment from contact with the major social institutions, as home, work, school, recreation, transport, or health care (a descriptor primarily of social health but may be tied to psychic and somatic capacities).

Internal satisfaction Enjoyment of living, self-fulfillment, or self-realization (a descriptor which is essentially psychic but which is likely to result from the degree of somatic or social well-being as well).

Adapted from H. L. Blum, *Planning for Health,* New York:Human Sciences Press, 2nd Edition, 1981.

distinctive amalgam of sensations, memory, knowledge, values, beliefs, imagination, and concepts which gives the person individuality, as well as an element of unpredictability to others, even to one's-self.

B. Psychic Health

Although systems logic forbids the fractionation of the individual's health into somatic, psychic, and social elements, there are some momentary advantages in doing so.[21] Psychic health is considered first because of its distinctive and central role in the functioning of members of the species *homo sapiens.*

Unlike other species, humans presumably have the capacity not only to be aware, but to know that they are aware, of most significant derangements of their sub-systems. This occurs when a person "feels" differently, as when one perceives pain, lassitude, functional failures, or when one senses that he or she is failing to receive expected messages through his or her own sensory equipment. By using sensory devices developed at the community level, such as laboratory analysis, the person also may test many of his or her own tissues, fluids, or sub-system activities for evidence of atypical states. One's introspective and contemplative will to observe his or her state of functioning, and one's response to these observations, are part of his or her psychic health. Thus, the person remains the servant of primal desires, no matter how much one's overt behavior is determined by supra-system or socio-cultural demands placed on him or her.

The person also has the innate capacity to store not only the prescribed guides of one's supra-systems, but to manufacture information, concepts, beliefs, and values, and to use those designed and stored by others. One is therefore able to generate new stances and influence others, as well as being influenced by them. The person may, as an individual or as part of a group, imagine or create visions of futures which may guide or move him or her even more than his or her sociocultural traditions. It is from these psychic visions that great religious and political movements are created. The interfacing, directing, and judgmental capacities of the person are also part of one's psyche.

It is apparent that a high proportion of day-to-day private, as well as public, legal judgments about the health of a person's psyche are primarily based on the perceived social appropriateness of one's behavior. This is not so remarkable, because how appropriately a person reacts to his or her supra- and sub-systems not only dictates the harmoniousness of their interplay but often determines one's survival as a person. However, this is far from being a suitable basis for judging psychic well-being, on two scores. First, when acceptability of behavior to peers is taken as the *sine-qua-non* of psychic well-being, one fails to take notice of serious, but still limited, departures from well-being that do not affect gross behavior. For example, modest euphoria, depression, anxiety, or unjustified worries, without grossly visible behavioral changes, still represent psychic aspects of systemic malfunctioning. Second, when psychic illness is arbitrarily limited to situations with gross behavior disturbances, some of us may be led to the idea that mental illness is a myth and that it exists only because society is seeking control of its social deviants by psychic labeling.[22]

The separation of psychic from social malfunctionings on one hand, and from somatic ones on the other hand, has been artificially-inspired by independent development of very narrow concepts which grew out of significant observations and interpretations (discoveries), at different periods, in cultures with differing beliefs, value schemes, ways of making people sick, and survival needs. Intellectual reconciliations became a necessity, and labeling became a means of bridging from one designated area of malfunctioning to another. For example, when a person's affect or behavior is seen as inappropriate *vis a vis* society, it may be called psycho-social illness. Correspondingly, when one is perceived to be interacting or responding inappropriately by placing unusual stresses or demands on one's sub-systems, the resultant condition is often called psychosomatic or psycho-physiologic illness.

But labeling also may lull us into overlooking the basic incompatibilities of limited conceptions. We are then led to ignore the real problems created by artificial boundaries, which impose limited and often highly inappropriate choices of interventions to be applied to malfunctioning at the so-called social, psychic, and somatic spheres.

Historically, perceptions of psychic health have varied widely over time and with cultures.[23] Perhaps the most widespread and indigenously occurring beliefs about psychic health were the "primitive" beliefs about the interrelatedness with nature of all social, somatic, and psychic manifestations of well-being. Long laughed at, this ecologic view is, of course, the precursor to the systems view of the world to which we are returning. The interveners called for by ancient ecologic views of health had to cover all bases with limited tools. They often used a mixture of interventions, some designed to alter a one's soma or physical sub-systems, others to alter one's psychic or integrative ones, and many to deal with one's supra-systems or social ones.

Let us glance at current modes of intervention used by those who provide psychic help, because their methods help us grasp the extent of the labeling dilemma and the conceptual limitations that need to be overcome. We can begin with Freud and the traditional psychoanalysts, whose work might be described as a direct attempt to put the psychic house in order. Freud sought to create better control at the conscious level by informing and aligning it with the more hidden levels of psychic forces. He recognized the utility of psychic interventions for many somatic maladies, and the social origins of many psychic and somatic disorders.

Other psychotherapists intervene primarily in the person's supra-systems, to stem their psychically-unsettling effects or alter them in ways calculated to restore the person's psychic balance (social therapy). Some seek to alter the disturbed person's environment only to the degree that there is less opportunity for one's aberrations (which go untreated) to clash with the modified environment.

Other psychotherapists utilize somatic or organic therapy, such as electro-shock, and achieve success with certain kinds of psychoses. Some somatically-applied interventions, such as Yoga or Rolfing, are not primarily directed to therapy of disorders but to promoting higher levels of somatic, psychic, and social well-being.[24]

The use of mood- and behavior-altering substances may be considered as somatic-level applications to alter psychic- and social-level functioning. How and where psychotropic substances really work is dubiously understood. Whether "favorable" alterations are to be regarded as social control, promotion of well-being, or as a therapeutic attack on deviance is not our concern here, except to point out that interventions or artificially-induced perturbations at one system level have the capacity to cause desired (as well as undesired) significant effects at other systems levels.[25]

The development and growth of an admittedly-eclectic school of psychotherapists provides further evidence of increasing awareness that interventions directed at the social and somatic systems, as well as directly at the psyche, are effective for some conditions in some individuals. In this view, it is a matter of refined case-by-case judgement to find the probable sources of perturbations and design the most suitable type of intervention to apply.

C. Social Health

Social health has been hard to conceptualize, yet deviations from it, such as role failures, are certainly among the most common events of concern to every culture. The state of a person's social health can be defined as the degree of appropriateness of one's behavior with the individual members of his or her family, with one's family as an entity, and with the hierarchy of *homo sapiens* systems which provide the instructions, persons, and other species with which the person must interact. The person who alienates self from family to hoard resources for him- or herself or progeny, who clear-cuts forest and silts and dams-up rivers, who destroys other species for pleasure, who strip-mines without regard to restoration, or who threatens directly the survival of others is demonstrating social ill-health. If the person is aware that one is prejudicing one's own future, or that of offsprings, by such ecologic rapacity, his or her social ill-health is simply more extreme.

In a society such as ours, which is undergoing rapid change and spawning sub- and counter-cultures, as well as being infiltrated by many persons from other cultures, it is rapidly becoming harder to settle on any suitable perspective from which to make judgments about social health. To further complicate matters, the same behavior viewed from different cultural bases may be identified as quite healthy, psychotic, or antisocial. These issues will be addressed when we scrutinize society's attempts to define health and illness.

Personally-destructive social behavior is expressed by such behaviors as driving at dangerous speeds and consuming excessive food, drink, tobacco, and drugs. Even when unperceived as hazardous, the commercially-promoted and socially-approved standards of behavior, which focus on enjoyment-to-the-hilt of the fruits of affluence, are obviously elements of social ill-health in one sense, even if socially-conforming in another. When the hazards are perceived and the destructive behavior continues, the phenomena may be based on psychic as well as social ill-health. The confusion of what is "good" for us, versus what makes us "feel good," may in itself be an important source of individual social and psychic stress.

Aging is now often seen as social illness. As the result of normal aging, persons cannot carry out the role activities expected of them at earlier stages of their maturation. In the eras and places where extended families occur, the usual capacities of the aging are seen as sensibly defining their role assignments, and they are kept at such tasks and are perceived as socially-useful and healthy. But where older persons are left in isolation, they cannot be an integral or useful part of a family system. As a consequence, they are thrown upon the higher supra-systems, such as the community, for support. The community in recent times has minimal use for their limited labors and experiential wisdom, particularly now that traditional wisdom seems less helpful than ever. Also, the community more often needs to reallocate the tasks formerly carried out by the aged to make jobs for unrelated younger people. In such societies, the aged become deviants, or socially "sick," when they are no longer self-supporting. Thus, the pressures of rejection and neglect are added to further deteriorate the normally-declining levels of social, psychic, and somatic functioning of the aging.[26]

Aging is normally associated with altered feedback, less homeostatic reserve, and less sub-system control. By definition, these are somatic and psychic failures if they are unthinkingly compared to performance at younger ages. By such mislabeling, we add further social pressures to hasten psychic and somatic failures, all of which we are taught to fear and avoid rather than to expect and tolerate. Even death is no longer seen as a normal outcome, but as an intolerable ending.[27]

D. Somatic Health

Somatic health encompasses the functioning of the sub-systems contained by the person-system level. We have already discussed anticipated variations in capacity that occur as a result of maturation and aging. Leaving these aside momentarily, any disruptions of physiologic function or anatomic integrity are regarded as somatic health failures irrespective of probable underlying factors or causes. Bodily discomfort, whether associated with somatic changes or not, must be accepted as somatic failure unless it can be placed among the psychic disruptions. Disease, of course, may occur without any awareness, but may be detected by specific testing or by testing the extent to which various homeostatic systems can keep reasonable equilibrium under calculated stresses. There is even an earlier stage of disease detection. Genetic scrutiny can often be used to predict the ultimate occurrence of a clinically-evident disease, such as diabetes. Genetic testing is also useful in determining diseases in a subsequent generation, as when a perfectly well carrier of sickle-cell trait can be told what the likelihood is of having a child with the disease if one marries a person with the same trait. The genetic status of an individual might be used to define the person as "sick" or "well," before or shortly after birth.[28]

If we are guided by a reasonable definition of health, such as *a state of being in which the individual does the best he can with the capacity he has and acts to maximize his capacities,*[29] a somewhat different set of standards must be applied to health. Currently, however, the expected effects of aging (or the consequences of somatic damage), such as skin keratoses, achlorhydria, presbyopia, cataracts, worn-out joints, osteoporosis, or conduction deafness, are classified as ill-health because they can be corrected or overcome, or their consequences can be ameliorated by one or another means. In other words, the standards of function to which somatically-damaged persons can be restored now defines the levels of health which can be anticipated, and anything less than that is considered ill-health.

The individual's dependence for good somatic health on a properly-interacting hierarchy of sub-systems, is attested to by a review of any of the well-understood somatic disruptions. The more we understand about why these failures occur, the more we have been able to ward them off. The more we understand about how these failures act, the better we have been able to supply missing parts or filter off or counteract harmful outputs. We even substitute artificial systems for ailing ones.

Some failures begin with hereditarily-transmitted defects which may prevent certain cells, tissues, or organs from developing appropriately. Other hereditary abnormalities work by means of disrupting metabolic pathways which, in turn, affect various bodily systems adversely by depriving, overwhelming, or poisoning them.

Various environmental impositions on the conceptus, such as infections, chemicals, or radiation, also produce specific damage on one or another level of inorganic or organic sub-system, thereby setting the stage for prompt or delayed development of somatic failures. Intrauterine-acquired (congenital) syphilis may cause serious prebirth organic damage, as well as delayed major damage in the ocular and nervous systems which may not surface for ten or 20 years. German measles, acquired early during the life of the fetus, causes major life-threatening multi-system defects. Some chemicals act similarly. Thalidomide causes phocomelia, an absence or distortion of limbs. Diethyl stilbesterol during pregnancy causes vaginal cancers in offsprings ten to 20 years later. The resultant somatic outcomes of intrauterine insults may be produced as a consequence of anatomic or functional failures of one or more specific cell, tissue, organ, or organ systems. Some failures disrupt the homeostasis of major systems and may be quickly disruptive or fatal. Some may only be activated at later stages of development or exert their abnormality-producing effects slowly. Nonetheless, once homeostatic mechanisms of one or many systems get beyond customary limits, sickness intervenes in the form of spreading disruption to more and more systems and leads to illness, incapacitation, or death of the person.

After birth, the person continues to be host to the various adverse hereditary and fetal environmental forces already set in motion. But, in addition, one is increasingly exposed to all kinds of new infections and chemicals, as well as to bouts of deprivation or excesses of necessary caloric, mineral, vitamin, protein, and other inputs. These are delivered in accordance with the person's location in the biosphere and in each of the supra-systems which embrace him or her. These supra-system controlled forces are omnipresent and their effects are overwhelmingly-interrelated. For example, malnutrition is key to the invasion and damage capable of being inflicted by infectious agents. Similarly, as indicated in **Figure 2.2**, disruptions or changes in value hierarchies or in political, social, economic, and other supra-system variables can lead directly to somatic damage, as by traumatic, chemical, or radiation injuries from war, traffic, employment, air pollution, and water pollution. More subtly, these same supra-systems can be the origin of unemployment, fear, social isolation and deprivation, excessive expectations, ego threats, and other pressures that just as surely end up disrupting the somatic systems in the *homo sapiens* hierarchy.

The continued use of the artificial distinctions of social, psychic, and somatic, laboriously raised between various manifestations of person-level system dysfunctions, are capable of doing us serious disservice except for their capacity to point up major conceptual disagreements on the nature of health. The two subject areas which follow try to make such disagreements more meaningful, and try to reveal the explanatory utility of the general systems paradigm presented in this book.

E. Spread and Apparent Transmutation of One Form of Ill-health Into Another

The ease with which dislocations in the supra-systems can pass from one to another, and to the person-level, is made clear by the example of a change in outlook on **war** versus **peace**, as shown in **Figure 2.2.** Significant perturbations among levels of the person's supra-systems are likely to result in maladapted behavior or responses which are social ill-health. (However, as has been noted earlier, perturbations ultimately may exert a positive effect in that they promote greater resistance, resilience, or growth and, thus, better health). At the same time, a person's social illness is likely to continue its wave of perturbations, so that one is unable to carry on suitable intrapersonal integration and therefore becomes emotionally ill. The ripples of disturbance may pass down into the somatic areas as well.[30]

The ease with which the person can disturb the supra-level systems is equally clear, from the example of a mutant resulting from radiation, as shown in **Figure 2.3.** Thus, whether being spread up or down, perturbations of any type, originating at any systems level, may result in disturbances of any kind: social, psychic, or somatic, or mixtures of all three. These occur typically in repeated episodes, whereby any combination of the three ill-healths are manifested in varying forms.

The significance of this dynamic state of affairs has never been seriously regarded by traditional therapists. The somaticists (most physicians) remove, repair, or adjust bodily parts and functions as though their handiwork were to last forever, even when it is grossly apparent that the causes of somatic illness are social stress, which, if left uninterrupted, will continue to further disrupt somatic systems. Some of the supra-system's social effects are direct. Lead poisoning occurs among neglected infants who ingest lead paint from walls of ghetto buildings. The lead poisoning is medically treated but often leaves irreparable damage, yet few effective moves are made to interfere with infant neglect, lead-painted walls, ghetto buildings, or social institutions that drive people to make and use such paint, live in such buildings, or neglect their children. Thus, the transmutation of one form of ill-health or deviancy into another is not only unremarkable, but routinely expected.

Remediation of socially-perturbed systems is particularly complicated, because many of our destructive socio-economic arrangements are socially devised and are also the source of our jobs and of our overall affluence. These arrangements liberate us from even more effective causes of illness and death that would operate if we were to remain in the underdeveloped state. With growing awareness that our blessings are far from optimal, we could alter our values and shift from an unrealistic and limited goal of increased survival of the affluent to a *survivial of the wisest.*[31] But survival in a state of wisdom, as seen by Salk, requires comprehension of the necessity to acknowledge and act on the inevitability of a now-beginning long phase of plateauing population, economic growth, and resource exploitation, or alternatively face recurrent booms and subsequent die-backs. Wisdom requires curtailment of the exuberant, exponential life styles and outlooks that *homo sapien's* journey on the first half of the signoid, or 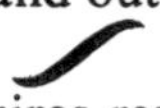 shaped, growth curve has given us. Survival wisdom currently requires restraint, decreased use of resources, living in moderation, and holding reproduction to near replacement levels. Even McHale and Cordell, who hold no brief for gainsaying the endless marvels to be expected from technology, emerge with a similar credo of required wisdom.[32] They find that the explosive growth of our future-altering, physical, technological capacities demand a comparable growth of conceptual wisdom and social technological skills. Without this wisdom, we cannot order or manage the changes we create and they, therefore, will blindly, and probably destructively, manage us.

These new wisdoms will undoubtedly require major alterations in present-day political forms built along the exploitive lines of capitalism, socialism, communism, fascism, and feudalism. It will be to the means of acquiring such wisdom, in regard to well-being and survival, that I direct many suggestions about how health-promoting services should operate.

F. Society Defines Health and Illness, and Designs Interventions Accordingly

Since maturation is a determining force in human existence, a definition of good health or capacities for functioning at one age cannot automatically be applied at others.[33] And there is wide variation in health among individuals at any stage of development. As a result, each society undertakes to define what is "normal" health at each stage of maturity in accordance with those capacities needed for the roles and tasks expected of each person.[34] Dubos says this differently: *Biological success in all its ramifications is a measure of fitness, and fitness requires never-ending efforts of adaptation to the total environment, which is ever changing.*[35] Since these definitions arise out of what the individuals in each society must successfully produce and what they must cope with, being healthy also varies from one social class to the next, from one place to another, over time, in any one place. Sedgwick makes an eloquent argument that the supra-systems, especially society, define all person-level system dysfunctions and determines whether they are to be labeled social, psychic, or somatic.[36]

Each society develops its own notions about the phenomena of ill-health, and dictates how the victim should behave, when one should suspect illness, how threatening one should regard it, and to whom he or she should or can turn for assistance.[37] In most societies, the person suspected of being ill is turned over to designated experts who are adjudged as capable of verifying the presence of, diagnosing the nature of, and prescribing therapy for the illness. In many cultures, verified sickness provides the victim with socially-accepted excuses for failure in various of one's roles or assigned duties.[38] More recent evidence enlarges such simplistic ideas and suggests a much more self-determined role for the sick person.[39]

Obviously, an integral part of defining illness and the behavior befitting the sick is the development of theories and procedures for diagnosis and treatment, as well as for training and directing those who care for the ill. These definitions vary with appreciation or beliefs about the origins of illness and how it can be averted or counteracted. The selection of honored, often feared, and occasionally heavily-sanctioned individuals, as carers of the sick, almost inevitably leads to class distinctions, approved modes of entry into the class of healers, development of societally-specified attributes for, and "licensure" of, healers to practice in one or another area of illness. With the growth of knowledge about bodily systems, subspecialization grows, and in Western medicine organizations or unions of practitioners are generally given the authority to define their own education, roles, and limits, even though almost always subject to nominal governmental affirmation or ratification. In fact, government generally undertakes to enforce the professionally-promulgated strictures. The boundaries and relationships of the ensuing maze of health professions are incredibly confused and complex.[40]

The designation of psychic, social, and somatic healers into spearate professional categories seems suitable only so long as there is little appreciation of the inseparability of psychic, social, and somatic health. The governmental imposition of new roles for healers in China highlights another aspect of the intertwining of social and somatic concerns, because it is a recognition that self-determined roles for healers might result in little valid or relevant care for the mass of a populace. For example, practitioners of all levels of expertise have been expected to provide significant periods of first contact or primary care out in the community. At the same time, candidates for training, in many cases of health care practice, are selected by the communities in which they work and to which they are expected to return. Equally interesting is the current Chinese political way (social, in our systems view) of treating the emotionally disturbed.[41] Those adjudged ill may receive extensive sessions with friends, family, co-workers, and professional health workers about the nature of their feelings and the consequences, and about their obligations to themselves and society.

Discussion of society's role in defining illness, the sick role, and the role of carers of the sick, can be further studied in several excellent works.[42] The resistance and reactions of healers to changes in their ways of serving society make equally-interesting reading.[43] This is further confounded by the turf-engendered professional separation of somatic from social and psychic concerns, which has probably led to a diminishment of humanistic responses from highly technologically-oriented practitioners. In the face of a broader comprehension of health by the public, there is a predictable patient rejection of non-caring responses from such providers. In turn, many of the providers see such wholistic searchings as an expression of anti-intellectualism against medicine.[44]

Some forms of illness and illness behavior are seen as law-breaking by societies, although healers may perceive them to be healthful attempts at survival by systems under pressure. Nonetheless, healers are required to report these behaviors to the police. Also, healers may place moral interpretations on various illnesses. Either state of affairs is likely to estrange healer from client and both from society, thereby preventing successful use of relevant interventions.[45] The difficulties facing persons who see health differently than do the accredited healers can also be imagined. The recent growth of new life styles has supported the development of new social organizations, such as "free clinics," many of which attempt to reconcile ways of healing with differing beliefs about the origins of illness and the nature of health.

These impasses illustrate the need for a more clarifying view of the nature of health that will bring the healers, the sick, and the well closer together in their efforts to promote well-being. I believe the general systems view begins to do so. Such studies as are built on observations of people at work and at play have long tried to attract our attention to the inseparable psychic, somatic, and social aspects of health.[46] More recently, the World Health Organization, through what has been called its "thoroughly impractical" definition of health, has given us an indication that the larger society is again expecting us to view health in terms of systemic interrelationships and general well-being.[47]

G. Aging, Natural Death, and the Compression of Morbidity

Using the title which we have borrowed from Fries,[48], we feel that it is important to draw attention to what could well be one of the most important changes in how society may shortly be viewing health, aging, and death.

By re-examining available data, Fries has made the discovery that we are eliminating needless premature disease, impairment, and death. At the same time, the **life span** of mankind does not seem to change after all. What does change is the average **life expectancy.** In fact, as societies prosper they sweep away needless or avoidable premature casualties. And as our resource capacities increase, we can sweep away more hazards. Thus, more of us are left who can reach our full life span which, in fact, seems not to change at all. Once said, this hardly seems strange, for every encyclopedic treatise on living things typically provides a statement of the usual life span of the species under discussion. Why should the life span of *homo sapiens* be indefinitely expandable if other species, much more easily juggled, are not? Yes, genetic engineering might do the trick of changing life span by creating a new species, *homo extendibilis.*

Fries and Crapo go further and point up that while increased societal safety nets can spare us from random casualties, we can at the same time redirect our living styles so that we maintain an improved level of youthfulness or plasticity.[49] By plasticity they mean that the future capability for a given human attribute "is not fixed, predestined or inevitable, but may be modified." Thus, use and strengthening of an attribute — physical, mental, or social — can be effectuated and a higher level of functioning maintained.

Notwithstanding, as we go through both a more hazard-free and a more healthy set of living activities, we still come to the end of the same old species life span. To use their analogy, a wise and well-spent life will terminate all of piece, just as did the one-horse shay. The delight of this logic is the optimistic cast it gives to increased survival. We are not being pushed into an increased life span, just a more healthy one, and one to which more of us live. And at the end of the road, a relatively short and less costly termination is envisioned, as all bodily systems begin to fail and there is little allurement or logic for replacing any one or two failing systems when all the others are also going or gone.

The following **figures,** taken from Fries and Crapo, provide a quick synopsis and data base which supports their most welcome theorizing. **Figure 2.5** illustrates the increasingly-rectangular curve of survival. **Figure 2.6** shows the minimal change in life expectancy at the higher ages and shows how the average life expectancy or survival is approaching the life span, but not adding to it. **Figure 2.7** illustrates the constant life span suggested by **Figures 2.5** and **2.6**. **Figure 2.8** shows that more life can be lived, i.e., at more vigor for a longer time, even though it does not affect the life span.

III. A PRAGMATIC SUMMATION OF FORCES THAT AFFECT HEALTH

For purposes of facilitating our ability to deal with the factors that affect health, it has been found very helpful to segregate the factors into utilizable groupings.[50] **Figure 2.9** boils down the myriad of systems' influences into four sets, which lend themselves to the analytic and synthesizing tasks facing anyone who desires to plan for better health. This I call the **Force-field Paradigm.**

The probable relative importance of the four aggregates of forces that have the major effects on health are portrayed by the width of the four input arrows shown in **Figure 2.9**. Clearly, the largest aggregate of forces resides in the person's environment. One's own behavior, in great part derived from one's experience with one's environment, is seen as the next largest force affecting health. Medical care services have been segregated out from the environment because of our great interest and investment in them. They make a modest contribution to health status. The contributions of heredity to health are harder to judge, but there is no doubt that we are templated at conception as to our basic weaknesses and strengths. However, many hereditary attributes never come to fulfillment because of the omnipresent environmental and behavioral forces which act before many genetic forces come to maturity. Many hereditary attributes are, of course, increasingly being palliated by medical care.

FIGURE 2.5
APPROACHING THE RECTANGULAR CURVE

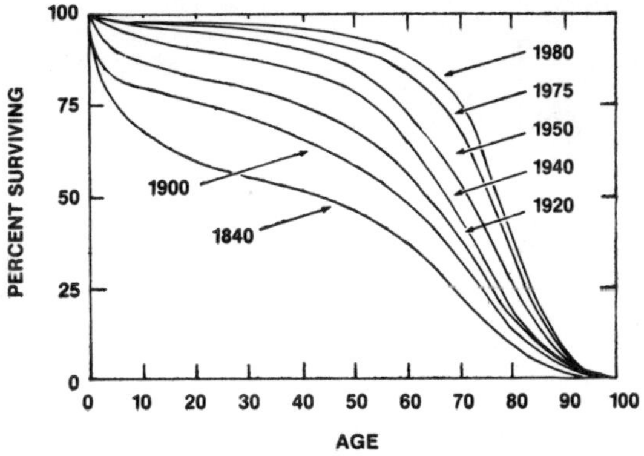

Sequential survival curves in the United States. The progressive elimination of premature death allows these curves to begin to approximate the curve that would be found in the absence of any premature death. (U.S. Bureau of Health Statistics.)

Taken with permission from J.E. Fries and L.M. Crapo, *Vitality and Aging*, San Francisco, W.H. Freeman, 1981.

FIGURE 2.6
CHANGES IN LIFE EXPECTANCY AT DIFFERENT AGES

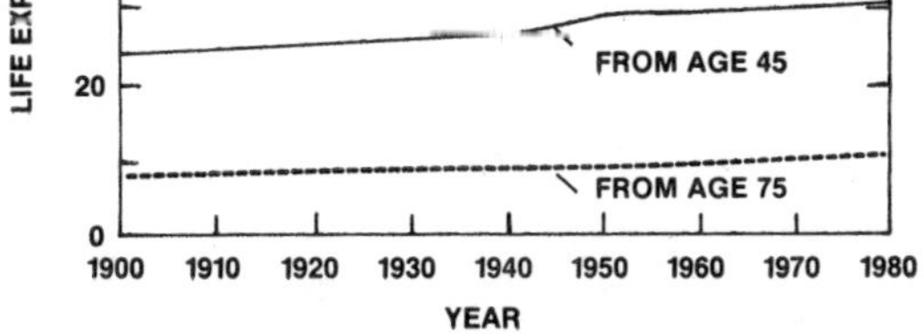

Changes in life expectancy in the United States during the twentieth century. From birth, life expectancy has risen from 47 years to 73 years. In contrast, from age 75, the increase has been only from eight years to 11 years. The greater the age from which life expectancy is calculated, the less has been the improvement. (U.S. Bureau of Health Statistics.)

Taken with permission from J.E. Fries and L.M. Crapo, *Vitality and Aging*, San Francisco, W.H. Freeman, 1981.

FIGURE 2.7
THE UNCHANGING LIFE SPAN

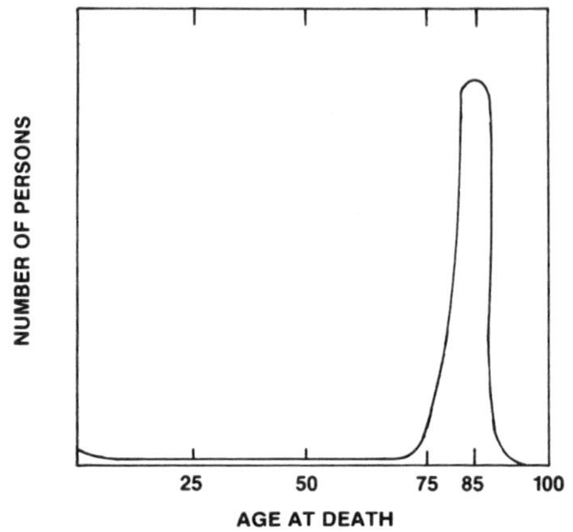

Ideal mortality curve in the absence of premature death. The average death occurs at age 85, with a standard deviation of about four years. Ninety-five percent of all deaths occur between the ages of 77 and 93. (U.S. Bureau of Health Statistics.)

From *Vitality and Aging: Implications of the Rectangular Curve*, by J. F. Fries and L. M. Crapo. W.H. Freeman and Company, Copyright 1981.

FIGURE 2.8
INCREASING FEASIBILITY OF A MORE VIGOROUS LIFE

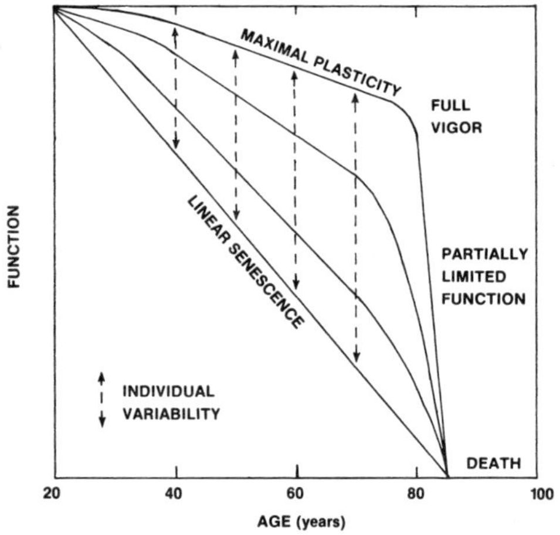

The individual rectangular curves for vigor, representing a lifetime of vigor followed by terminal collapse.

From *Vitality and Aging: Implications of the Rectangular Curve*, by J. F. Fries and L. M. Crapo. W.H. Freeman and Company, Copyright 1981.

The peripheral ring of the diagram makes the point that the four major forces are related to one another and affect one another through their mutual dependency on what might be called the key sub-strata, e.g., natural resources, ecological balance, population, cultural systems, and human satisfactions.

The centrum of the figure, the object of our concerns, is health. It is represented as an encompassing state of inseparable and transmutable aspects of psychic, social, and somatic well-being (which, unfortunately, in

FIGURE 2.9

THE FORCE-FIELD AND WELL-BEING PARADIGMS OF HEALTH

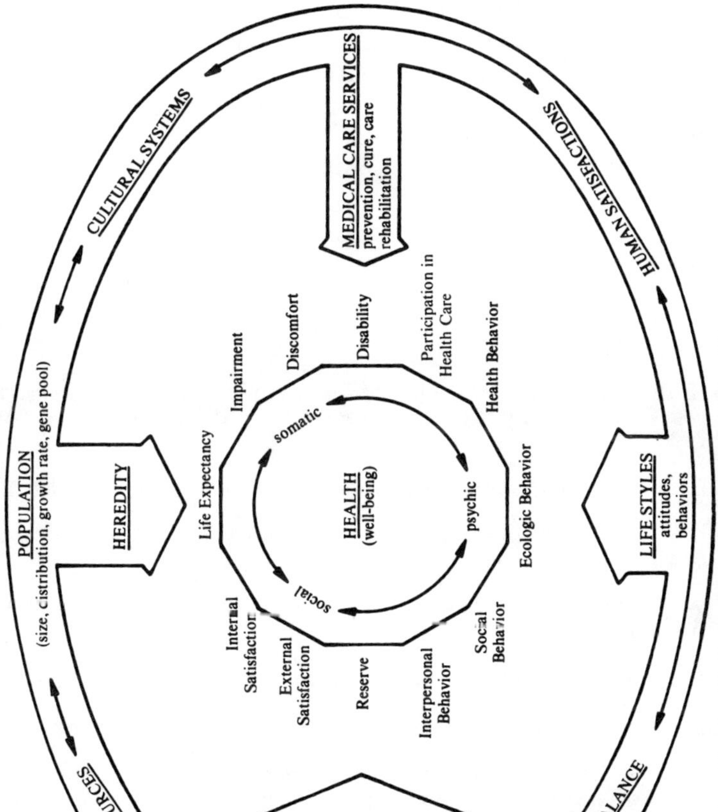

Adapted from H. L. Blum, *Planning for Health*, Human Sciences Press, N.Y., 1981.

western cultures, have been regarded as separate entities). This I call the **Well-being Paradigm.**

It should be noted that throughout this text the terms holistic or wholistic are generally avoided, even though it would seem that the two paradigms encompassed in **Figure 2.9** embrace essentially all of the concepts introduced under the rubric of wholism. This avoidance is not accidental. Wholism has come to mean many things besides the wholeness or oneness of well-being.

More likely than not, when confronted with a self-styled "disciple" of wholistic health, one can generally anticipate that the disciple will be antitraditional medical care, often even excluding it from consideration. This is not what wholistic means to me. I have in mind the systemic interrelatedness of all relevant contributions to good and bad health, and for all the possible interventions, traditional or not, that can be brought to bear to improve health and that are directed at any level of the hierarchy of systems that we have examined.

REFERENCES

1. H. Brody, "The Systems View of Man: Implications for Medicine, Science, and Ethics," *Perspectives in Biology and Medicine,* 1973, 17:1, (Autumn), 71-92.

2. E. Laszlo, *The Systems View of the World,* New York, Braziller, 1972.

3. L. L. Cavalli-Sforza and W. F. Bodmer, *The Genetics of Human Populations,* San Francisco, W. H. Freeman and Co., 1971, 39.

4. W. Buckley, *Modern Systems Theory for the Behavioral Scientist,* Chicago, Aldine, 1968, 490-513.

5. A. Koestler, *Janus,* New York. Vintage, 1978, Appendix 1, 289-311.

6. D. Speer, "Family Systems: Morphostasis and Morphogenesis, or Is Homeostasis Enough?", *Family Process,* Vol. 9, Number 3, September, 1970, 263-273. E. Wertheim, "The Science and Typology of Family Systems II, Further Theoretical and Practical Considerations," *Family Process,* Vol. 14, Number 3, September, 1975, 286.

7. A. Kuhn, *The Study of Society: A Unified Approach,* Homewood, Ill., The Dorsey Press, Inc., 1963, 38-54.

8. H. Brody, Ibid No. 1.

9. B. B. Brown, "New Mind, New Body," *Psychology Today,* 1974, August, 45-

112. E. E. Green and A. M. Green, "Regulating Our Mind-Body Processes," *Fields Within Fields,* 1973-4, 10 (Winter), 16-24.

10. H. T. Odum, *Environment, Power and Society,* New York, Wiley Interscience, 1971, 58-59.

11. C. C. Delwiche, "The Nitrogen Cycle," *Scientific American,* 1970, 223:3, 137-146. J. McHale, *The Ecological Context,* New York, Braziller, 1970, 53-55.

12. L. R. Brown, *Seeds of Change: The Green Revolution and Development in the 1970's,* New York, Praeger Publishers, 1970.

13. "Green Revolution I: A Just Technology, Often Unjust in Use," *Science,* 1974, 186:4169, 1093-1096. "Green Revolution II: Problems of Adopting a Western Technology," *Science,* 1974, 186:4169, 1085-1088. F. M. Lappe, "The World Food Problem," *The Hastings Society Studies,* 1973, November 11-13.

14. *WHO Chronicle,* "Is There a Protein Problem?" 1973, 27, 487-491.

15. P. R. Jennings, "Rice Breeding and World Food Production," *Science,* 1974, 186:4169, 1085-1088. A. Mayer and J. Mayer, "Agriculture, the Island Empire, " *Daedalus, Proceedings of the American Academy of Arts and Sciences,* 1974, 103:3, 83-95. R. Rodale and T. Dybdahl, "The Coming Food Crunch," *Cry California,* 16:3, Summer 1981, 6-12.

16. B. Commoner, "Alternative Approaches to the Environmental Crisis," *Journal of the American Institute of Planners,* 1973, 39:3, 147-162. T. Farvor and J. P. Milton, *Careless Technology,* Natural History Press, New York, 1972.

17. H. Brody, Ibid, No. 1.

18. H. Brody, Ibid, No. 1.

19. P. Sedgwick, "Illness — Mental and Otherwise," *The Hastings Center Studies,* 1973, 1:3, 19-40. R. M. Veatch, "The Medical Model: Its Nature and Problems," *The Hastings Center Studies,* 1973, 1:3, 59-76. *WHO,* The International Classification of Impairments, Disabilities and Handicaps, Geneva, 1981.

20. H. L. Blum, *Planning for Health,* New York, Human Sciences Press, 2nd Edition, 1981, 14. S. Fanshel and J. W. Bush, "A Health Status Index and its Application to Health Services Outcomes," *Operations Research,* 1970, 18, 1021-1066. S. B. Goldsmith, "The Status of Health Status Indicators," *Health Services Reports,* 1972, 82, 212-221. J. D. Hennes, "Measurement of Health," *Medical Care Abstracts,* 1972, 29, 1268-1288.

21. C. B. Bahnson, "Epistemological Perspectives of Physical Disease from the Psychodynamic Point of View," *American Journal of Public Health,* 1974, 64:11, 1039-1040.

22. T. S. Szasz, *The Myth of Mental Illness,* New York, Hoeber-Harper, 1961.

23. "Facing Death," *The Hastings Center Studies,* 1974, 2:2, 2-80. M. Foucault, *Madness and Civilization: A History of Insanity In the Age of Reason,* New York, Vintage Books, 1973. I. Illich, "The Political Uses of Natural Death,"

The Hastings Center Studies, 1974, 2:1, 3-20. G. Rosen, *Madness in Society,* London, Routledge and Kegan Paul, 1968.

24. A. Lowen, *The Language of the Body,* New York, Collier-MacMillan, 1971.

25. R. Neville and others, "Controlling Behavior Through Drugs," *The Hastings Center Studies,* 1974, January, 2:1, 65-112.

26. *Annals of the American Academy of Political and Social Science,* "Political Consequences of Aging," 1974, 415, 1-212.

27. Ibid, No. 23.

28. M. Lappe, "Genetic Knowledge and the Concept of Health," *The Hastings Center Studies,* 1973, 3:4, 1-3.

29. H. L. Blum, Ibid, No. 20.

30. A. Slote, *Termination: The Closure of Baker Plant,* Indianapolis, The Bobbs-Merrill Co., 1969.

31. L. R. Brown, Global Witness, *Rockefeller Foundation, Illustrated,* 1974, 2:1, 3. M. Mesarovic and E. Pestel, *Mankind at the Turning Point,* New York, E.P. Dutton and Co., 1974. J. Salk, *The Survival of the Wisest,* New York, Harper and Row, 1973. J. Salk and J. Salk, *World Population and Human Values,* New York, Harper and Row, 1981.

32. J. McHale and M. Cordell, *World Trends and Alternative Futures,* Honolulu, East-West Center, 1974.

33. E. H. Erikson, *Childhood and Society,* New York, Norton, 1950, 247-269.

34. T. Parsons, "Definition of Health and Illness in the Light of American Values and Social Structure," in E. G. Jaco (Ed.), *Patients, Physicians and Illness,* Glencoe, The Free Press, 1958, 165-187.

35. R. Dubos, *Mirage of Health,* New York, Harper, 1959, 25.

36. Ibid, No. 19.

37. Antonovsky, "A Model to Explain Visits to the Doctor: With Specific Reference to the Case of Israel," *Journal of Health and Social Behavior,* 1973, 13, 446-454. J.T. Shuval, *Social Functions of Medical Practice,* San Francisco, Jossey-Bass, 1970.

38. T. Parsons, *The Social System,* Chicago, Free Press of Glencoe, 1951, 428.

39. E. Freidson, "Client Control and Medical Practice," *American Journal of Sociology,* 1960, 65, 374-382. E. Freidson, *Patients' Views of Medical Practice,* New York, Russell Sage Foundation, 1961. E. Freidson, "Disability as Social Deviance," M. B. Sussman (Ed.), *Sociology and Rehabilitation,* Washington, D.C., American Society of Sociologists, December 15, 1965, 71-99. E. Freidson, *Profession of Medicine,* New York, Dodd, Mead and Co., 1970. E. Freidson, *Professional Dominance,* New York, Atherton Press, Inc., 1970, Chapter 1. D. Hayes-Bautista, "Patient and Practitioner: The Interaction of Assessments," Mimeograph, University of California, Berkeley, 1974. D. Mechanic, "Health and Illness in Technological Societies,"

The Hastings Center Studies, 1973, 1:3, 7-18. J. Roth, *Timetables,* New York, Bobbs-Merrill Co., 1963. M. Siegler and H. Osmond, "The 'Sick Role' Revisited," *The Hastings Center Studies,* 1973, 1:3, 42-58.

40. R. Roemer, "Social Regulation of Health Manpower," in *Fostering the Growing Need to Learn,* Division of Regional Medical Programs, Bureau of Health Resource Development, PHS, DHEW, Rockville, Md., 1974. Commission for Alternative Systems of Medicine, "Alternative Medicine in the Netherlands," *World Health Forum,* 1982, 3:2, 204-208.

41. V. W. Sidel and R. Sidel, "Medicine in China: Individual and Society," *The Hastings Center Studies,* 1974, 2:3, 23-26.

42. F. N. Arnhoff, "Social Consequences of Policy Toward Mental Illness," *Science,* June 1975, 188:4195, pp. 1277-1281. M. Foucault, Ibid, No. 23. Ibid, No. 39. T. Mann, *The Magic Mountain,* New York, Vintage Books, 1969. D. Mechanic, *Medical Sociology,* New York, The Free Press, 1968, Chapters 3, 4, 5. Ibid, No. 37. Ibid, No. 38. Ibid, No. 19. H. E. Sigerist, *A History of Medicine,* New York, Oxford University Press, Vol. 1, 1951, Vol. II., 1961. *The Hastings Center Studies,* 1973, 1:3, 3-88. Institute of Medicine, *Community Oriented Primary Care,* Washington, D.C., National Academy Press, 1982.

43. E. Cray, *In Failing Health: The Medical Crisis and the AMA,* The Bobbs-Merrill Co., Inc., Indianapolis, 1970. P. de Vise, "Misused and Misplaced Hospitals and Doctors, Commission on College Geography Resource Paper No. 22," *Association of American Geography,* Washington, D.C., 1973, 51-57. R. Stevens, *American Medicine and the Public Interest,* New Haven, Yale University Press, 1971.

44. R. H. Moser, "An Anti-Intellectual Movement in Medicine," *Western Journal of Medicine,* May, 1975, 122, 433-449.

45. R. C. Allen, "The Insanity Defense: An Uncertain Future," *Mental Health,* 1974, 58:4, 4-7. J. Satten quoted in R. C. Allen, "The Insanity Defense: An Uncertain Future," *Mental Health,* 1974, 58:4, 4-7.

46. I. H. Pearse and L. H. Crocker, *The Peckham Experiment,* New Haven, Yale University Press, 1946.

47. D. Callahan, "The WHO Definition of 'Health'," *The Hastings Center Studies,* 1973, 1:3, 77-88.

48. J. F. Fries, "Aging, Natural Death and the Compression of Morbidity," *New England Journal of Medicine,* 303:3, July 17, 1980, 133.

49. J. F. Fries and L. M. Crapo, *Vitality and Aging,* San Francisco, W. H. Freeman and Co., 1981.

50. H. L. Blum and Associates, *Notes on Comprehensive Planning for Health,* Western Regional Office, American Public Health Association, San Francisco, October 1968, School of Public Health, University of California, Berkeley, 3.02-3.03. H. L. Blum, *Planning for Health,* Human Sciences Press, New York, 1974, Chapter I. H. L. Laframboise, "Health Policy: Breaking the Problem Down Into More Manageable Segments," *Canadian Medical Association* Journal, 1973, 108, 388-393. M. Lalonde, *A New Perspective on the Health of Canadians,* Government of Canada, Ottowa, April 1974.

Chapter 3

EVIDENCE SUPPORTING A GENERAL SYSTEMS OR ECOLOGIC VIEW OF HEALTH

Robert G. Robinson* and Henrik L. Blum

Evidence supporting general systems logic can be placed in the four useful, although not mutually exclusive, categories shown in the force field on **Figure 2.9,** page **37**. Examples have been selected in each category that help explain how perturbations at various levels of systems create significant amounts of human illness. The studies referred to under "Utilization of Scientific Medicine" shed light on the significance of medical or somatically-directed therapy in the preservation or restoration of health, as well as the far-from-minimal adverse effects of modern therapy (iatrogenicity).

Historic trends provide remarkable insights into the probable causes of the waxing and waning of the frequency and severity of various human illnesses. In spite of generally poor recording of health events, many countries provide us excellent chronicles of the frequency of death, even by probable cause of death. These can be correlated with the historically-associated patterns of living, working, eating, and care for illness.

Nearly all of the great infectious scourges of the Dark Ages and Middle Ages had almost disappeared by the time their etiology, prevention, or therapy had become understood.[1] Their disappearance or their

---

*At the time of this writing, Mr. Robinson is a candidate for the degree of Doctor of Public Health, School of Public Health, University of California, Berkeley.

lessened invasiveness or destructiveness is ascribed to generally better living conditions, and particularly to suitable nutrition, clean food and water, better education, safer employment, and more compatible general environment, including safer and more protective housing. In the U.S., for example, the downward path of the mortality trends for tuberculosis, from 1900 to the present, was interrupted briefly by the social cataclysms of World Wars I and II. It is clear that anti-bacterial or anti-disease treatments had little to do with the drop in mortality rates.[2]

At the same time, other diseases, not of the clearly contagious sort, such as deaths from cancer of the stomach, have also shown a long-term decline in no way relatable to medical care. Other diseases, also without useful medical interventions, have had a marked rise in mortality. In association with increased air pollution and tobacco smoking, there has been a spectacular rise in lung cancer and emphysema. Apparently, as women pursued equality they took up smoking, and their pulmonary disease pattern is now following right along on the heels of that for men.[3]

In England and Wales, life expectancy at age 45 had not improved significantly between 1870 and 1970.[4] In the U.S., life expectancy at birth in 1900 was approximately 47 years, while in 1979 it was 74 years. However, at age 65 in 1900, it was 12 years, while in 1979 it was only 17 years, showing that the gains had been made primarily at the younger ages and reflected, in particular, the sparing of infant deaths.[5]

The retrospective glances just reported on, and others to follow, make clear the folly of ascribing massively-favorable or unfavorable changes in health status to single or directly causative sequences of events, such as the interventions of medical care. Under medical care, we will have the opportunity to examine the remarkably favorable results that treatment of hypertension has had in the downward overall death rates in the U.S. over the past 15 years, results that are probably due more to avoiding the consequences of hypertension than from preventing it. Further encouragement is justified for improved health status or at least quality of life from scientific efforts, such as inexpensive and allergy free insulin, drugs, and surgery to alleviate arthritic pain or coronary artery damage, a vaccine for hepatitis, new techniques for treating cancer, and skin regeneration for burn victims. However, the prognosis generally for improved research and development in the pharmaceutical field is not altogether favorable.[6]

Even more has been anticipated from changes in life style and from improving the environment, particularly as it affects life styles. However, as Fries and Crapo say so well, we can and may well increase our **life expectancy** as much as ten years by cutting into the premature deaths. However, what we do know indicates that we will not increase the average **life span** of *homo sapiens* beyond age 85.[7]

Unfortunately, one is entitled to deep concerns evolving from the understanding that health status will be dictated more by the mechanisms of *homo sapiens* supra-systems. The increasing homicide rates for our young adults, or the increasing world populations and decline in per capita resources, are not reassuring to the citizens of any country. Perhaps the most relevant example is the potential pathology and death stemming from "the last epidemic," a function of society's reliance and faith on nuclear energy and weapons as primary means of living and problem solving.[8] The data do give us every reason to believe in the major consequences for human health from the rise or decline of perturbations in the supra-systems high in the *homo sapiens* hierarchy of systems.

I. CORRELATIONS OF WELL-BEING WITH SPECIFIC ECONOMIC, SOCIAL, CULTURAL, AND PHYSICAL ENVIRONMENTAL VARIABLES

The pursuit of supposed cause-and-effect relationships that seem to explain the incidence, prevalence, and distribution of specific diseases and illnesses in a given population is the work of epidemiologists and ecologists. It has led to intensive comparative study of sub-groups, illustrating how various factors present in one group, but absent or diminished in another, can be said to be **independent** variables determining a range of conditions or outcomes which are called **dependent** variables. Many key leads about the causes of good and bad health have been learned from such comparative population studies, despite the plethora of pitfalls inherent in study design due to the limitations of naturally-occurring "experiments," cross-sectional analyses, and unreliable data bases. The state of the art demands an ongoing critical assessment of research. We accept, for example, the correlation of prevalence of high blood pressure, coronary heart disease, and cancer with social class, minority status, sex, age, personal habits, and, simultaneously we appreciate the complexity as well as value of such searches.[9] New discoveries will be shaped by the appreciation of how history influences the recognition and interpretation of data;[10] a broadening and refined view of causality in the etiology of disease;[11] a strengthening of the ecological model;[12] a growing emphasis on environmental factors and the idea that social structural forces and a generalized susceptibility to disease underpin much morbidity and mortality;[13] and a growing awareness that scientific methodology is evolving into a new paradigm, influencing our world-view and perspectives of etiology.[14]

A. Poverty, Affluence, and Race

The poor suffer poorer health, by all traditional measurements (primarily somatic), and large groups of them (primarily minorities) are often further disadvantaged by not receiving appropriate services and by obtaining less care.[15] The general conclusion is of an inverse relationship existing between socio-economic status and health when the health status indicators are overall morbidity and mortality.[16] Furthermore, and regardless of what modifications might occur in the definition of status, all evidence shows the lowest segment of a society has the greatest burden of morbidity and mortality.[17] Indeed, when compared to other socio-economic variables, income is a factor which increases in importance particularly at the deepest levels of poverty.[18] In general, poverty is associated with greater persistence of negative health.[19] Comparison of poverty and non-poverty areas show poverty areas adversely affect health, even when social status is controlled.[20] Life seems particularly hard for blacks in the aggregate, regardless of where they live. The overwhelming weight of evidence also shows a correlation of psychiatric illness with social status.[21]

The implications of these correlations are reinforced because poverty in the U.S. deepened during the seventies. The hardest hit are minorities and women, with poverty in the central city actually increasing after 1969. Indeed, a sensibly-modified version of the "official poverty definition" would increase the percentage of poverty in the population from 11 percent to 21 percent, from 30 percent black families to 45 percent, from 35 percent female-headed households to 50 percent, and finally, from 50 percent among black female-headed households to 70 percent.[22] Black mortality was higher than whites, in 1977, for every age group, particularly ages 25-44 where mortality was 2.4 times greater and, in addition, age-adjusted deaths in the U.S., except for suicide, were higher for blacks than for whites.[23]

There is a remarkable correlation between the incidence of tuberculosis and poverty among white males in various age groups. There is also significant correlation between poverty and cancer of the stomach in white men and women. It is also twice as high in men as in women at all economic levels.[24] The incidence of stomach cancer, regardless of economic level, is higher for black males and females, with the mortality rate for them, in 1973, twice that of whites. The rate of decrease for both incidence and death since 1947, due to stomach cancer, favors whites of both sexes.[25] Overall, the decline of stomach cancer since the thirties, compared to the ten percent increase of all cancer incidence in the decade (1968-1978), is most striking.[26]

Racial comparisons of incidence (1947-1969) and mortality (1950-1973) of all cancer sites indicate that non-white males have undergone the greatest change, and are at greatest risk.[27] Mortality for non-white females, compared to white females, was higher in 1950 and 1973. Mortality for non-white males was lower in 1950 and higher in 1973, compared to white males. The percentage change of mortality for black males, from 1950 to 1970, was a phenomenal 63 percent increase.[28] Site-specific data indicate dramatic increases in prostate cancer for black males,[29] large increases of lung cancer for black males and females, increases in lung cancer and melanomas for white males and females, increases of prostate, bladder, and kidney for all males, and a sharp decrease in cervical cancer for women.[30] A relationship between social status and melanoma mortality for females, and incidence levels for males and females, is indicated.[31]

The age-adjusted rates for morbidity and mortality of cardiovascular diseases has been declining at least since 1968, with coronary heart disease (CHD) mortality decreasing 24.3 percent from 1968-1978,[32] and cerebrovascular artery disease or strokes by 40 percent. These two declines account for most of the total death rate declines in the U.S., and for closing the gaps between white and black mortality, as blacks had a greater gain.[33]

Relationships of prevalence of heart conditions (CHD, rheumatic fever, rheumatic heart disease), cerebrovascular diseases, stroke, and hypertension were inversely related to levels of income and education in 1972.[34] Hypertension, in particular, has been studied extensively, and a relationship to social status is indicated for morbidity and mortality.[35] Similarly, the prevalence of hypertension, and levels of blood pressure, are higher among blacks for every age group[36] except among the children and adolescents. There is evidence that when social status is controlled, race is no longer significant.[37] Populations experiencing particular historical oppression have higher blood pressure levels.[38] Consistent with blacks' disproportionate mortality for hypertension, is evidence indicating that they experience more severe degrees of organ damage[39] and poorer control status.[40]

Age-adjusted mortality for heart conditions and cerebrovascular disease historically have been higher for blacks, and remained so in 1975.[41] Coronary heart disease, comprising the large majority of heart conditions, was higher for whites after World War II, but the gap has since reversed for black females and has almost closed for black males.[42] CHD is particularly ominous for blacks, due to the higher rates of CHD mortality at younger ages. It is this age-specific difference which makes CHD the largest mortality cause among blacks, a phenomenon not often noted because of the increased percentage of excess deaths of blacks, compared to whites, from other causes, particularly from stroke and violence.[43] A strong social-class relationship with CHD is found in England, with a higher rate of mortality found in the lower classes.[44] In fact, grade-of-employment proved a stronger predictor of CHD than any other risk factor.

Prevalence of diabetes in 1973 was higher for blacks, particularly ages 45-64, and was related to income for this same age group. It was related to education for all age groups. Age-adjusted mortality from diabetes mellitus, historically, has been higher for non-whites, particularly among non-white females compared to white females.[45]

Significant correlations between low family income and high post-neonatal mortality, and low birth weight, have almost never failed to be verified, and infant survival bears remarkable relationships to socio-economic variables, even after effects of medical care have been controlled.[46] Neonatal and post-neonatal mortality have declined.[47] From 1960 to 1978, the decrease was approximately 45 percent, yet the relative position of the U.S., compared to other western countries changed but little. Among the 16 top industrialized, non-communist countries, the U.S. was tenth in infant mortality in 1960, while in 1978 it was 11th and tied with three other countries.[48] In 1980, the U.S. continued to gain, but our rate of 12.5 was evidently still behind ten other countries that had lower rates in 1978 than did the U.S. in 1980. Infant mortality and low birth-weight ratios for blacks is twice the white rate.[49] A most impressive relationship of well-being to economic factors is shown by infant death rates in the U.S., which respond to levels of economic adversity as measured by unemployment.[50] The same correlation between economic instability and infant mortality has been observed for England and Sweden. Infant mortality is also higher in poverty areas.[51] It is obvious that income and infant mortality are complexly related; when mortality is high, the relationship is in great part apparently-dependent on patterns of living associated with relative deprivation, poor education, and cultural patterns.[52]

Malnutrition and poor nutrition (generally, but not always a consequence of poverty) have been specifically identified as critical factors in the predisposition to, and outcome of, infections, and a pervasive influence in determining infant and early-childhood morbidity and mortality.[53] The relationship between malnutrition and infant mortality is also a function of social class.[54] Nutrition also has been repeatedly suggested as a critical factor in the development of the brain tissues in infants.[55] The problem is compounded, given the indication that rising food costs will divert low-income communities from foods high in nutrition, as well as by the likelihood that many of the mothers having to work for additional income actually add to the level of malnutrition in their infants.[56] Indeed, replacing the loss of breastfeeding, in terms of equivalent nutrients, can constitute 50 percent of the mother's earnings. A similar consequence was indicated in Britain where, because of higher rents for better housing, the diet of low-income families suffered and morbidity increased, despite the better surroundings.[57] The production and export of infant formula contributes an estimated million infant deaths a year in the Third World as a result of diarrhea and malnourishment associated with misused and contaminated formulas.[58] The interlocking web of malnutrition, infant mortality, and social class underscores the assessment that the solution is not increased production of food (equitable distribution of current food supplies are sufficient to eradicate malnutrition of children), better relief programs, or population control; rather, it is the resolution of income inequality and poverty.[59]

B. Economic Development and Fluctuation

It is considered indisputable by some that high blood pressure and cardiovascular disease are a product of modern class societies,[60] or from the industrialization of society.[61] Whether or not disease and mortality can be consigned to specific historical eras, there is evidence that epochs characterized by scarcity, or societies plagued with underdevelopment and homogenous scarcity, do not show correlations of class and health status.[62] A cross-sectional comparison of two rural communities demonstrated the effects of development. The health status of the "underdeveloped" village was significantly better than the "developed" village characterized by wage labor and migration.[63]

It is certainly possible that the health status of underdeveloped societies are adversely affected by the encroachment of external economic and political forces, leading to irrational development, and resulting in the distribution of health status by social status similar to developed societies.[64] There are several examples where the effects of encroachment result in the creation of wage labor, disruption of social life, migration, dietary changes, and population growth, and succinctly demonstrate how a relatively-healthy population can become diseased as a result of specific economic and political policies.[65] It is eminently clear that these patterns will remain unaltered unless dynamic changes are made in the economic and social structures of such societies. There are a few, but significant, examples whereby changes occurred at these levels and resulted in increased equity and improved health status.[66] In some cases, progress was reversed when the political environment reverted to its previous inequitable condition.

The dynamics of developed societies are different. What appears to affect post-industrial societies are the consequences deriving from the cyclical swings or fluctuations in the economy. Employment patterns, migration, inflation, rapid cultural change, loss of income, social relationships, and stress patterns emerge as key indicators predicting the effects of economic process and policy on health status. Thus, unemployment is directly related to an increase in infant mortality, deaths from heart disease and chronic nephritis, first admissions to mental hospitals, mental illness (loss of job can be the first step towards psychosis), alcoholism and cirrhosis-of-the-liver mortality, child abuse, suicide, homicide, and imprisonment rates.[67] Loss of job has been shown to permanently affect one's perception of the future and degree of optimism,[68] and to all forms of somatic, psychic, and social disruptions.[69]

It is possible that some specific diseases are directly responsive to economic upswings and others to recession. Consequences of the former are influenza, pneumonia, cardiovascular disease, strokes, cirrhosis and accidents; of the latter, they are suicide, homicides, crime, and mental illness.[70] The common link in each pattern is the relationship of well-being to economic processes and policies, and the need to analyze health-status changes historically in relation to economic development and the associated changes in social structure.

C. Education

Significant relationships have been shown for income and education to mortality and morbidity, generally, with education emerging as the better predictor.[71] Because education and economic status so closely parallel one another, as well as correlating with housing, employment, access to opportunities, age distribution, and so on, the effects of these variables are difficult to separate. In addition, there are particular problems with blacks, given the differential roles played by education and income in determining social status when compared to whites.[72] These differences emerge due to the distinctive cultural and historical contexts of the two races, and the pervasive influence of discrimination and institutional racism. Thus, it is confusing when variables such as education, occupation, and income have been standardized within predominantly-white communities.[73] Similarly, a problem exists when status has been calculated with the black segment of the population removed from the analysis.[74] Most importantly, equal educations by race do not lead to equal occupations or income by race.[75] The net result of such disparities will be to mis-estimate the social status of black people generally, mis-interpret the meaning of the status that is estimated, and mis-calculate the status differences of black people and between the races.[76]

D. Occupational Exposures and Job-related Health

The National Institute for Occupation Health and Safety estimated in 1972 that 100,000 persons die a year and another 390,000 become ill as a consequence of working in American industry. It is generally accepted that the true extent of these casualties is probably much higher than official tabulations indicate.[77] There are unlimited, documented episodes of every kind of occupational hazard, and their resultant diseases can be reviewed in several texts,[78] but the magnitude of the problem is not certain. Information is lacking, and relative risk is difficult to ascertain because of the complex interaction effects between exposure levels and other risk factors. It is generally accepted that more people are killed by slowly-developing occupational diseases than by work accidents.[79] It was estimated that one in four workers are exposed to hazardous substances regulated by the Occupational Safety and Health Administration (OSHA), and at least 50 million workers may have been significantly exposed to more than one hazardous substance at some time in their life.[80] Agricultural workers are at particular risk.[81]

Estimates of all cancers contributed by the workplace are ten percent to 38 percent.[82] One of the earlier and more tragic results of occupational exposure was scrotal cancer, which occurred in the waifs used as human "chimney brushes." It is estimated that, for the remainder of the 20th century, 17 percent of all cancer deaths may well be attributed to asbestos, for it is linked to cancer of the lungs, esophagus, stomach, colon, rectum, kidneys, pleura, and peritoneum.[83] Certain coke-oven jobs, in the steel industry, place workers with more than five years experience at 11 times the risk of lung cancer compared to other steel workers. Rubber workers, 40-64 years old, have three to seven times the risk of dying from lymphatic leukemia than the general male population. Atomic energy workers die at twice the rate from cancer of the pancreas than a comparable population.[84] Interestingly, persons with regular outdoor jobs are at very low risk for melanomas compared to indoor workers.[85] Factors operating here are assumed to be self-selection and the possibility of a sudden exposure mechanism underlying the etiology. Melanoma is believed related to chemical carcinogens in work sites.[86] The bladder cancer rate in New Jersey is the largest in the U.S., and is concentrated among white males.[87] Two factors must be noted: one-half of the U.S. chemical industry is located in New Jersey, and it utilizes skilled trades mostly limited to whites. Discriminatory employment practices also determine cancer outcomes. For example, 326 out of 496 coke workers studied by Lloyd were black.[88] Studies of rubber, agriculture, steel, textile, laundry and drycleaning, and shipbuilding and repair industries show significantly higher levels of cancer for black workers.[89] Discriminatory placements in the most hazardous jobs are the underlying causes. In addition, shift work, comprising 27 percent of all labor in 1975, typically not voluntary and therefore more likely for minority workers, is related to an array of physical and social symptomotology and disease.[90]

Women-on-the-job tend to be less protected than men, because most regulation is directed towards male-dominated labor. Nevertheless, employment places men at greater risk because of the higher ratio of hazardous jobs they undertake.[91] In general, working women, compared to non-working women, have a higher incidence of acute conditions, fewer chronic conditions and symptoms, better general health, and fewer days of bed rest or restricted activity. Sales workers have a higher risk of leukemia; office and clerical workers are subject to tenosynovitis; health care workers have higher risks of infections and backstrain injuries; and operating room personnel run a higher risk of cancer and spontaneous abortion due to exposure to various anaesthetics. Indeed, even the wives of operating room personnel have higher rates of miscarriage and birth defects.[92] Similarly, the wives of males exposed to vinyl chloride have higher rates of miscarriage and stillbirths; increased risk of angiosarcoma of the liver; and cancer of the lung, blood-forming tissues, brain, and central nervous system. Disturbances in the menstrual cycle occur among women involved in the manufacture of diethylstibesterol.[93]

The social ramifications stemming from our use of the adversary posture between employers and employees has had sad consequences.[94] Early laws, to provide off-setting awards to persons injured by or at their work, passed through a phase of determining if the worker had contributed to the problem, as by carelessness. Later, workmen's compensation laws provided awards that often served to deter use of preventive devices or of return to work. It is questionable whether labor has ever possessed sufficient control of the workplace to enable issues of health, rather than safety, to be primary. Also to be questioned is an emphasis on health that seeks to eliminate at-risk individuals from the workplace rather than addressing the causative basis for the health hazard.[95] Many current insurance practices dealing with the re-employment of disabled persons serve to prevent employment of those with suspected or known impairments or disabilities. The outcomes of such legal (social) constraints are highly associated with social, emotional, and somatic illnesses resulting from the stresses and barriers to survival that they occasion.

E. General Physical Environment

The physical environment is composed of a vast number of interrelating elements. Many of their effects can be separated only by the cleverest of controlling devices and data manipulation. However, these will be considered individually whenever there are useful data.

1. Housing, crowding, and population density Crowding in homes (dwelling density) apparently has very little effect on well-being and "deeper" emotional levels, even though such things as worry and unhappiness increase, particularly when crowding is with non-kin.[96] Crowding was also considered less important for mental health than forced interaction with another household sharing the same unit. Lack of options to escape the environment may also be a factor.[97] Crowding is felt to be less important than population density in increasing pathology, general hospital admissions, morbidity, and social maladaptation.[98] Population density, with crowding as a component, proved less important than social structure, with status as a component, to age-specific rates of psychiatric admissions.[99] Crowding is described as a possible factor in higher blood pressures in Taiwan, West Africa, and prison settings.[100] Perception of crowding in prison settings had no effect on blood pressures for blacks or whites.

Significant health changes were not demonstrable in a controlled study of families moving from dilapidated to modern housing.[101] By contrast, the hazards to infants, in poor homes with lead paint, are all too clear. This has been verified for children living in census tracts defined as low status.[102] Similarly, accident rates are considerably higher in bad housing. The supposed higher rates of infection among crowded poor people may be more dependent on effects on individuals resulting from limiting space or territory between individuals than on the increased ease of transmission of infectious agents. The crowding theories of contagious disease spread have been deflated by showing that when education and income are controlled for, the contagious disease-housing correlations disappear.[103] The point has also been made that it is often the terrible health status of the bottom social class that allows a class difference to be shown for chronic diseases. This is an important observation, for many other deleterious forces are probably acting in concert in that bottom group. Dilapidation, poverty, and ignorance may account for the apparent importance of housing.[104]

2. Air pollution The relationship of air pollution to well-being is demonstrated by its relationship to asthmatic attacks, bronchitis, emphysema, and lung cancer.[105] More long-term and indirect is the relationship of air pollution to stomach cancer and its variance by sex and economic class, which can be postulated as the result of forces affecting the degree and extent of exposure.[106]

There is a consistent relationship between ventilatory function in children age five to 13 years, and exposure to particulate matter plus sulfur dioxide. Heavily-exposed children also improved in seasons with lower pollution, but not to levels of function exhibited by children in neighborhoods with cleaner air.[107] A positive relationship exists between quantity of particulate matter suspended in air and mortality and morbidity of heart disease, as well as for mortality in general.[108]

There is no evidence that urban living *per se* is related to occurrence of respiratory diseases, thus pointing to air pollution as a significant factor in its own right.[109] Sulfur dioxide levels provided a consistent predictor of mortality in New York.[110]

There is evidence that a reduction of 60 percent in urban air pollution can be expected to reduce pulmonary cancer by 20 percent in every category of tobacco smokers.[111] Airborne carcinogens are synergistic with alcohol and tobacco.[112] Mortality from asthma, bronchitis, emphysema, and lung cancer are higher in urban areas than rural.[113] There is good evidence that childhood lead poisoning is nòt solely a phenomenon of ill-cared-for children ingesting lead paint, but is also dependent on inhalation of lead-containing, automobile-exhaust fumes.[114]

3. Traffic The dangers of highways are clearly correlated with correctible hazards. A curve-correction program is credited with a 67 percent reduction of accidents and a 55 percent reduction in injuries and fatal accidents. The effect of lessened use of alcohol can well be imagined, because the association of high alcohol-blood levels and accidents is a remarkable one. The 1973-74 energy shortage, which resulted in modestly lessened traffic and slightly slower speeds, had a major effect on the frequency of accidents. Mortality due to traffic accidents is higher for non-whites than whites. Interestingly, age-specific data show that black youth, ages 16-24, compared to white youth, have fewer traffic accidents, which presumably results from their lack of access to cars and licenses.[115]

4. Noise Correlations between noise and well-being suggest a meaningful interaction. Long-term exposure to occupational noise has been said to raise one's risk of cardiovascular disease by 60 percent. It is related to mental hospital admissions, with persons most at-risk being the single, widowed, and separated. Noise does not appear to increase mental illness; rather it aggravates existing psychological problems. Noise can interfere with psychological and cognitive development at home and in school, and is believed to have an effect on the cardiovascular, endocrine, respiratory, and digestive systems; and it increases blood pressure. Experiencing aircraft noise contributes to mortality from strokes, cardiovascular, cirrhosis, lung cancer, suicide, and auto accidents. High-level noise in the military or industry is definitely related to hearing loss and a temporary shift in the threshold of hearing. Noise reduces a person's sociability and degree of sensitivity to the needs of others. Significantly, a person's attitude and belief about the sound may mediate the affects of noise and be more important than the intensity.[116]

F. Stress

Although the use of the word "stress" is not always favored because of its ambiguous usages, sometimes in the sense of describing stressors (forces or system perturbations imposing on an individual), sometimes as the physiologic alterations which result from such forces, and sometimes as the symptoms which can result, it still seems to be an invaluable concept.[117] Density, sociologic stressors, and psychic pressures will be briefly explored as aspects of stressing.

1. Population or areal density As indicated in the section on housing, population density is interactive with crowding, the quality of social interaction, and, as such, it is difficult to separate its effects. Nevertheless, there is good evidence that areas with increased population density have more tuberculosis, pneumonia, chronic disease, disability, suicide, infant mortality, mental illness, and venereal diseases.[118] Consistent with the finding in Hong Kong, in relation to crowding, lack of territorial control may be a factor of more significance.[119] However, conclusions must be made cautiously, given the correlation of these outcomes with so many other factors which also correlate with population density.

2. Sociological stressors The term "sociological stressors" represents an increasingly-complex set of interrelated forces that can be expected to affect all aspects of well-being. The substance of stress is not easily defined, particularly since the range of indicators used to represent it has been so vast. Work is needed in terms of theory and operationalization to more clearly allow an understanding of the etiology between "stressors" and well-being. Stress may even be that mild bane of sociologists, a matter of simple common sense.

One of the easiest somatic disturbances to measure is elevated blood pressure. Elevated blood pressures and hypertension-related mortality repeatedly occur with increased variety and severity of stressful living conditions (often represented by social disorganization).[120] Similarly, dark skin color for blacks was related to increased blood pressure, in addition to suppressed hostility. Dark skin color was not a factor in whites of Mediterranean heritage.[121] The probability that psychosocial factors mediate between skin color, hostility, and blood pressure must be a consideration, particularly when controlling for social status produced no association between skin color and high blood pressure.[122] Stress, it would appear, must be viewed as part of a context if it is to be understood. More coronary disease and mortality have been reported among mobile than stable people.[123] This suggests that a kind of stress response is made by people who either "don't fit" or who are in strange environments. The latter reflects the importance of social support systems. Increasingly, social support systems, social networks, and the quality of social interactions are appearing to be relevant in the mediation of stress and well-being, as well as in constituting a determining effect in their own right (see support networks).[124]

More heart disease is reported in stable rural people in neighborhoods that are undergoing rapid change than in neighborhoods remaining unchanged. There is evidence that wealthier blacks in a white area have more tuberculosis than blacks in the ghetto. There is evidence that residents of new suburbs experience more emotional disturbances among women and children, have more hospitalization for depressive disorders and for suicide, and have a different pattern of psychosomatic illness. Those who are a "good fit" with the dominant types in their environment experience fewer problems.[125] Stresses of the "don't fit" variety suggest that the "loss of biologic buffers" calls for new sources of feedback, such as friendship, support, trust, and appreciation.[126] Animal experimentation supports such conclusions. Rats shocked in isolation developed more ulcers than those shocked in the company of their litter mates. Mice also develop more hypertension if they are forced into a transgressor role.[127] The relevance of the social support concept is evident.

Enforced relocation, such as that experienced by the residents of Boston's West End, was associated with significant grief reactions in this tightly socially-knit group.[128] It is also well known that the elderly in nursing homes do worse after relocation to "better" environments, presumably as a result of the stressing arising from loss of familiar settings, persons, and activities.[129] Similarly, mortality is increased for those moving to nursing homes, particularly in the first year.[130] In general, stress events are linked to incidence of tuberculosis, clinical depression, anxiety, schizophrenia, heart attacks, chronic asthma, respiratory diseases, streptococcal infections, complications in pregnancy, and skin diseases.[131]

Stress on the job produces several outcomes. Persons who do not have control of the workplace, who do not have correct qualifications for their job, or who experience conflicting demands, have higher blood pressure than those who do not have these problems.[132] Lack of a good job, not only loss of a job, is related to crime. Also, social integration and stable employment are key variables mediating between high stress and psychological symptoms.[133] Lack of control of the work process, frustration, overwork, excessive demands, and responsibilities on the job are related to CHD.[134] The intensity of work frustration experienced at the onset of a heart attack and the degree of work-related problems experienced proved to be significantly related to recovery from a severe attack.[135]

3. Life Changes Such stresses have been divided into long-term and short-term, and both are significantly associated with increased illness. The consequences of such stresses affect individuals as well as family units, encompassing chronic illnesses as well as family breakdown. It is not necessary for the life situation to be negative; rather, the common thread appears to be one of "change." Changes might be the so-called socially favorable ones, such as getting married or getting a promotion, or the unfavorable ones, such as experiencing a family death, divorce, loss of a job, and so on. No one disease is associated with any one type or grouping of crises, but the more-severe diseases are associated with more-aggregate stress. Even the frequency and severity of football players' injuries were found to be correlated with intensity of stresses provoked by life changes.[136] Illnesses cluster, and the more episodes one individual has, the more kinds of illnesses he or she is likely to develop. In one study, those with exaggerated illness records not only had evidence of stressful childhood but felt they currently had a "bad" life situation. So, the stressed are more vulnerable, and have more troubles or ill-health of every kind. "Giving up," under more stress than can be tolerated, is thought to be a key first step or invitation to developing illness.[137]

II. CORRELATION OF WELL-BEING WITH BEHAVIOR AND LIFE STYLE

Control of present health problems in the U.S. will depend significantly on modification of individual behavior and habits of living.[138] It is a matter of strategical and philosophical debate whether the direction for these changes ought best emanate from political and economic policy or reside primarily in the realm of individual education and behavioral change (see **Chapter 4** for further discussion).

A significant association exists between health status and the amount of sleep, erratic eating, alcohol consumption, weight, smoking, and regular exercise. The more of these factors that are bad, the worse the health status.[139] At the extreme, the health status of persons who scored well in every area were similar to persons 30 years younger who scored poorly.

A. Smoking

Smoking is related to moderate anomalies in infants, to CHD, and to cancer of the lungs, mouth, pharynx, larynx, esophagus, and urinary bladder.[140] The World Health Organization identifies smoking as the single-most important perturbation affecting health and mortality in all of preventive medicine. It is the largest contributor to cancer mortality, larger than all other risk factors. Smoking, along with the concommitant phenomenon of the tobacco industry as an integral component of the economy, is cited as a major underlying factor in CHD rates, and is one of the larger contributors to the phenomenal increasing mortality rates in the Soviet Union.[141] In the U.S., the proportion of male smokers from 1965 to 1979 decreased from 51 percent to 37 percent, and of females from 33 percent to 28 percent.[142] The percentage of black males who smoked was more than for white males, but rates were similar for females. However, blacks smoked on average a fewer number of cigarettes than the number smoked by whites.[143] The prevalence of smoking is increasing among the young, particularly females, and helps to explain the climbing incidence of emphysema and cancer among women.[144] Similarly, the lower lung-cancer mortality of Mexican-American women, when compared to white women, is explained by the different prevalence of smoking in each population.[145] The economic gains from the tobacco industry were estimated to be less than $12 billion, while the costs for the health consequences were estimated to be $18 to $27.5 billion.[146] Several findings indicate that neither the increase in percentage of black smokers nor the overall decrease of smoking in the population explain the patterns of CHD mortality.[147]

B. Diet

Diet and obesity are related to blood pressure, heart attacks, atherosclerotic diseases, and strokes, to cancer of the gastro-intestinal tract, to diabetes, to liver and gall bladder disease, to degenerative arthritis of the hips, knees, and ankles, and to injuries.[148] Eighty-five percent of children who are obese become obese adults. A critical factor is the increased number of fat cells, via infant feeding, during the third trimester, one-two years of life, and pre-adolescence.[149] Suitable alteration of the diet is estimated to reduce cancers by 35 percent. Ironically, polyunsaturated fats (puf) increase the risk of cancer while also decreasing the risk of CHD.[150] Serum cholesterol levels are significantly lower in countries where the puf intake is high.[151] Two hundred mg/dl is considered a threshold for serum cholesterol in populations, and if the U.S. were to reduce to this level, a 15 percent decrease in CHD is estimated.[152] Vegetarians have been shown to have less hypertension and, also, decreased risk of cancer.[153] Unfortunately, there are findings to indicate that fat intake and cholesterol levels do not explain patterns of CHD mortality.[154]

C. Alcohol

Alcohol is related to accidents, to cirrhosis, to vitamin deficiencies, to inflammation of the pancreas, esophagus and stomach, to muscular and neurologic diseases, and to cancer of the mouth, pharynx, larynx, and esophagus.[155] The percentage of cancers associated with alcohol varies from 6.1 percent to 9.1 percent for whites, from 11.3 percent to 12.5

percent for blacks, and the highest is 27.9 percent in Puerto Rico.[156] The percentage of persons considered to be heavy alcohol users and who also develop cirrhosis of the liver is 61 percent to 89 percent. Cirrhosis has been correlated with state policies regarding sale and distribution of alcohol.[157] England, during World War I, increased alcohol taxes and lowered availability of time for selling alcohol.[158] Subsequently, cirrhosis liver mortality dropped from 10.3 per 100,000 population in 1914 to 4.5 in 1920. The tax increases remained in effect after the war, and mortality continued to decrease to 3.1 by 1936. In the U.S., wartime prohibition decreased cirrhosis mortality from 11.8 to 7.1 in 1920; it was still 7.2 in 1932, the year before prohibition ended. But following repeal, and without a restrictive tax policy, cirrhosis mortality increased to 16.0 in 1973. The percentage of deaths due to automobile accidents associated with alcohol is 50 percent to 75 percent and 11 percent of all deaths are directly or indirectly related to alcohol.[159]

D. Exercise

Low physical activity has been strongly associated with increased prevalence of heart disease.[160] Moderate exercise is popularly associated with fitness and a general state of well-being.

E. Manifest Health Behavior

Manifest behavioral patterns often integrate personal knowledge, life style, health care utilization determinants, and the availability of primary intervention; and consequently are often related to educational, economic, and social levels. Health-affecting failure in such behavior are associated with lessened health reserve and increased mortality.[161]

By mid-1979, 90 percent of children ages five to 14 had been immunized for measles, polio, diphtheria, tetanus, and pertussis, and 85 percent for rubella. But, in 1978, among children aged one to four, 38 percent were not immunized for rubella, 37 percent not for measles, 49 percent not for mumps, 39 percent had not received the recommended dose schedule for polio vaccine, and 32 percent were not appropriately vaccinated for diphtheria-pertussis-tetanus (DPT). Immunization levels for polio and DPT actually decreased from 1970 to 1978. Persons most likely not to be immunized were minorities, and children living inside central cities of standard metropolitan statistical areas.[162] The largest racial difference existed for polio.[163]

In 1973, after years of accepted use and intensive propaganda, only 57.4 percent of women ages 17 and over had had a pap smear in the previous two years; and, as expected, increased income was positively related to obtaining such testing.[164] In 1976, one-third of American women had never had a test, and of those who had it, one-third had not had it for six years.[165] The record is similar for electrocardiograms and glaucoma screening.[166] Education correlates with use of preventive services and is the best predictor of birth control and prenatal care.[167] The use of seat belts in cars and airplanes has been shown to reduce the risk of injury and mortality for both infants and adults.[168]

F. Support Networks

The absence of support networks has shown up for decades in the parade of statistics about the poorer health of widowed, divorced, separated, and single persons. In more recent times, it began to show up in several contexts, one of which we have already discussed as the ability to mediate stress. In other situations, it appears to have demonstrated a positive role of its own[169] (see **chapter 4**).

The parade of effects on health status by various environmental variables is an impressive one. There can hardly be any doubt about the massive and omnipresent effects on human health which are caused by perturbations in the supra-systems of *homo sapiens.*

III. CORRELATION OF WELL-BEING WITH GENETIC CONTRIBUTIONS

The particular intrinsic and hereditable nature of this determining force warrants specific treatment.

A. Maladaptation

We have learned to accept the fact that there is a markedly-increased incidence of degenerative diseases as societies industrialize. Even when race is controlled for, the differences between pre-industrial and industrial societies remain tremendous. Powles makes the point that *homo sapiens* made most of the species' biological adaptations over more than 50,000 generations, when activities and nutrition were continuously that of hunter-gatherer.[170] Only in the last 300-400 generations has *homo sapiens* become the effective agriculturalist or industrial worker. In recent centuries, changes have occurred with increasing rapidity, and significant groups of *homo sapiens* have left behind the environment to which they had become selectively adapted. In other words, *homo sapiens* has had little time or chance to mutate and selectively adapt to the new nutrition, types of exposures, and stresses.[171] Dominant diseases of industrial societies, such as arteriosclerosis, probably represent just such maladaptations.

B. Specific Conditions

At the disease-specific level, there is a mass of data that describes not only evidence of the genetic role in statistical terms but provides the specific genetic makeup of many disease conditions and their response capacity to environmental factors.[172] In fact, laboratory information is now so good for many specific conditions that we can determine whether the defect is dominant or recessive, whether it is based on full, excessive, or limited chromosome complement, whether it is on the sex determining chromosomes, or others, and whether it is of high or low penetrance (the degree to which the properties of a gene are evident).[173] The introduction of perturbing forces, in the form of medications for various conditions, has resulted in the "discovery" that there are many genetic makeups which preclude toleration or metabolization of one or another drugs.[174] Thus, another aspect of human adaptability is put on test with the intentional imposition of new interventions. "Failures" to tolerate drugs could also be classified as diseases.

C. Resistance to Disease

The inherited capacity to resist various conditions has been documented extensively.[175] But it has to be recognized that the final health outcome of the individual is dictated by the combined effect of internally-dictated (genetic) strengths and weaknesses and of forces from the environment that are relevant to bringing out these strengths and weaknesses.

The importance of the genetic constitution in determining health status cannot be doubted, but what is a favorable genetic configuration (e.g., sickle cell), in the face of one environment (sea level and malaria) may turn out to be a most unfavorable one in another environment (high altitude).

IV. CORRELATION OF WELL-BEING WITH THE UTILIZATION OF "SCIENTIFIC MEDICINE"

Because so many people, including scientists, erroneously equate health status solely with use of medical care, this latter force, an undeniably important one, has been singled out for more careful scrutiny. In spite of clear-cut clinical evidence regarding better survival from innumerable conditions after certain kinds of therapy, there is only controversial evidence that more and more scientific doctoring will be associated continuously with better and better health status or with increased survival.[176] In part, this is the case because most extensive doctoring is associated with diseases that are heavily associated with the aged, thus affecting a population who, despite being saved from one threat, are likely to succumb shortly to another. Moreover, a significant portion of doctoring goes for purposes that have little to do with extension of life or freedom from disease and its effects. Probably half or more of medical care is devoted to caring or treatment which may improve functions or overcome disability and freedom from discomfort, but which does not actually cure disease or restore health. What is more to the point is the potential price of care for people who are prematurely running down, and how the years of life can be given added vitality so that the normal life span of 85 years can be attained with better and safer living and a lesser load of premature chronic ill-health burdens.[177]

It is also true that much doctoring is associated with the shift of social service burdens to the health sector, as by putting frail elderly persons needing modest supervision and assistance into nursing homes. Also, much doctoring is used for societally-required certification, sorting, and institutional supervision: activities that are directed only minimally toward promotion of the recipient's well-being.[178]

A. General Availability and Utilization of Medical Care

When life expectancy in countries is compared with their expenditures for treatment, prevention, information, and so on, it is evident that as much as 86 percent of all the variation in health status of infants and children can be accounted for by the availability of potable water and literacy. The levels of medical care available are irrelevant to outcomes.[179] In developing countries, health care services will be ineffective until measures are taken providing for safe water supplies, adequate housing, improved nutrition, and sanitary waste disposal.[180] In the U.S., interstate variations in extent of medical services have been compared with mortality, and there is some correlation but it is not nearly as significant as the effects of income and education.[181]

B. Enhanced Utilization of Medical Care

There was no change in morbidity or mortality in a group of poorly-served persons who received comprehensive medical care over a three-year period, when compared with a control group.[182] Similarly, no difference was observed in morbidity or mortality in an experimental group of aged persons given high-quality medical care when compared with a control group which received poor and fragmented care.[183] In a Guatemalan setting, added medical care provided no measurable gain in terms of decline of episodes of illness.[184] Navajos, living in primitive circumstances but with adequate nutrition, had significant health improvements in only two types of sickness, middle ear infections and tuberculosis, as a result of adding good primary medical care.[185] When the treatment modalities emphasize village personnel, community participation, or alternative medical practitioners, rather than clinical care, the outcomes are appreciably more positive.[186]

C. Quality Control of Medical Care

In Britain, mortality for certain conditions has been observed to be lower in teaching hospitals.[187] This raises the possibility that adding medical care without controlling its quality may not reveal the true significance of relevant medical services. A broad view of quality will focus on the interface with the client and the medical care system, on how many clients are able to receive care, on the level of met needs, and on the optimal benefits for the individual and population. Given a broad view of health, quality of care is a function of the extent to which possible improvements in the quality of life are obtained as a result of that care. It is also possible that above some modest level of care, the impact of additional care of reasonable quality adds little to the ultimate well-being of a populace but a good bit of iatrogenicity. The main utility of quality control might therefore result from assuring freedom from activities of unrestrained entrepreneurs who use procedures needlessly, and from medical quacks (a restraint on quantity as well as quality).[188]

D. Addition of Specifically-relevant Medical Care to Selected Populations at Known Risk from Specific Hazards

The effectiveness of chemotherapy for victims of such infections as bacterial meningitis, septicemia, pneumonia, syphilis, tuberculosis, even leprosy, is outstanding.[189] However, long-term incidence trends also show that the spectacular decline (or increase) of such conditions, or of their severity, are also heavily a response to environmental changes and are quite independent of the availability of chemotherapy.[190] Chemotherapy remains primarily of significance to the individual cases that do occur.

Evidence of improved outcomes among coronary artery occlusion victims, when they were cared for in intensive care units rather than at home, is not satisfactory.[191] Given that there is evidence that anxiety is able to trigger further clotting,[192] it may be that home care more than offsets the anxiety that might be occasioned by the victim's removal to a hospital, and to subsequent exposure to the implied threats as well as to intensive care equipment and routines. Mobile coronary-care units have proven effective in sudden cardiac attacks.[193] Coronary-bypass surgery is effective in restoring pain-free functional capacity from severe coronary artery disease, although it is not clear that it significantly prolongs life as compared to medical regimes.[194]

The most exciting evidence of effective medical care in the U.S. is the continuing reduction of deaths from coronary heart disease (CHD) and cerebrovascular disease (strokes), manifested since about 1966. Almost the entire improvement in lowered death rates among adults is due to a decline in these two diseases, which are heavily the consequences of uncontrolled hypertension. No one will give the entire credit to pharmaceutical control of these diseases because of the decline in smoking among males, decreased fat intake generally, and increased exercise patterns. However, the remarkable changes of 24 percent decline in CHD and 40 percent decline in stroke from 1968-78 for black and white males and females, which are still continuing and are more pronounced among blacks, suggest improved chemical control as well as compliance with medical care, both of which we know to be taking place.[195] Some researchers have serious reservations about these conclusions.[196]

Another good example of effective health care intervention lies in the area of maternal and infant care projects.[197] The introduction of nurse-midwives and public health nurses decreased infant mortality of disadvantaged pregnant women.[198] Nutrition advice has been positively related with a decrease in prematurity rates.[199] Research projects in Guatamala, Nigeria, and the U.S. have demonstrated that primary care and increased nutrition substantially impact on mortality of infants and children, ages one-four, even if delivered by auxiliaries, with only limited referrals to physicians or hospitals.[200] The establishment of comprehensive care clinics for poor children resulted in a 60 percent decrease in rheumatic fever, when compared to children with similar demographic characteristics who were ineligible for the program.[201] Family planning and increase in abortions, as a result of legalization, have been associated with reductions in infant mortality rates.[202]

Several major studies show that there is significant risk to infants as a result of three kinds of factors: social, such as literacy or culture, demographics, such as race and age, and lack of medical care. Not only are maternal illiteracy and minority race real hazards, but so are obstetrical complications, which we know can be alleviated by skilled care. The risks go up as the patients have one, two, or three of the adverse factors. Prenatal care, when controlled for by race, is effective in lowering infant mortality. Low birth weight correlates better with infant mortality than any other variable.[203] Other factors responsible for affecting mortality include birth order, age of mother, maternal education, race, and legitimacy status.[204]

Poverty and bad living conditions correlate with low birth weight, but the use of medical care *per se* essentially has no effect on low birth weight. Lewis et al., who did a key study, conclude that *this is not to say that good medical care is not important, but rather that there may be forces of social and environmental origin that are more determinant in the long run. These forces, such as crowding, victimization, demoralization, malnutrition, and physical and emotional strain, all apply long before the pregnancy, apply more broadly than to the prospective mother alone, and are not something to be erased by medical care.*[205] What is hard to visualize is how much worse off these high-risk people would be without traditional one-to-one medical care.

It is possible to conclude that medical care directed to prevention or amelioration of specific conditions is increasingly effective, spectacularly so in some situations. What cannot be said is that increasing amounts of medical care, beyond some basic minimum properly targeted, is correlatable with any evidence of generally-improved well-being. Medical care, even when effective for correction of preventable conditions, is not always as wise an approach to improving health status as the utilization of feasible, preventive procedures. Prevention of lead intoxication or of poliomyelitis are both examples of feasible preventive approaches. Both are based on advanced scientific comprehension, but the former is entirely non-medical in application and the latter requires no skilled health workers to administer. It is also arguable that medical care is the victim of increased and unrealistic expectations.[206]

E. Hazards of Medical Care (Iatrogenicity)

The word **iatrogenic** means "illness caused by what the physician does or prescribes." Webster's unabridged *Third New International*

Dictionary offers *imagined ailments induced by autosuggestion based on a physician's words or actions during an examination.* Undoubtedly, this definition was coined a long time ago when one of the most tangible effects the pre-scientific physician could have was from the way of performing an examination or of discussing the condition with the patient.

In our use of the term **iatrogenicity**, we combine all inadequate or harmful outcomes in the patient as the result of interventions applied to others or to other species, as well as directly to the patient.

There are many aspects of iatrogenicity:

1. The patient pursues an unhealthy behavior pattern, because he or she has been ineffectively advised.
2. The patient is correctly treated by technical means consistent with the ailment, but is incorrectly treated in light of his or her functional and role needs, or psychosocial requirements.
3. The patient is correctly treated for one condition, but the therapy does harm to other unknown or unknowable conditions to which he or she is subject.
4. The patient is correctly treated, but the treatment causes a severe reaction in other tissues, such as depression of immunity.
5. The patient is incorrectly treated (or not treated) when he or she should be, and the condition remains unimproved or worsens, or new problems are created because of failure to halt the old one.
6. The patient's problem is not understood by the practitioner because of cultural differences, and the patient is essentially barred from appropriate care.
7. The patient behaves so that he or she interferes with, negates, or distorts therapy in a harmful way, irrespective of the technical correctness of therapy given.
8. The patient is the victim of changes induced in disease agents (e.g., invasive organisms that have become drug resistant as a result of specific therapy given to other persons) or is exposed to diseases in the medical care environment (e.g., nosocomial or hospital-acquired infections). Between them, these factors probably cause as many as 100,000 deaths in the U.S. each year.[207]
9. The person is unintentionally exposed (as in food or drink) to various substances intentionally used as medications or growth inducers or inhibitors in plants and animals, substances which have for the person all the properties and hazards (albeit unsuspected) of medications, or so alter the person that he or she cannot use or tolerate the same or

related interventions when needed.

10. The patient is incorrectly advised that he or she has a disease, and his or her life is needlessly altered as a consequence.[208]

It must be made clear that the removal of a limb for a hopeless infection, tumor, or injury is not considered iatrogenic, because this is the exact purpose of the therapy. However, if an infection were to develop as a result of surgery, or a phantom limb syndrome were to take over, these would be iatrogenic. Iatrogenicity does not *per se* suggest physician error or incompetence, for the physician and the patient may wisely agree to pursue a course of care in the presence of necessary iatrogenic risks having known and anticipated frequencies.

How important are iatrogenic conditions to society? Nader testified in December, 1973 that the Food and Drug Administration had stated that more than 100 Americans die daily as a result of reactions to legal or non-legal drug prescriptions.[209] It was estimated that 33 percent of the present volume of antibiotics are unnecessary, and approximately 2000 patients served by private office-based physicians die annually as a consequence of adverse antibiotic reactions.[210] A University of California staff conference pointed out that three percent of hospital deaths are drug related.[211] (The average hospital patient is said to be given six to ten drugs per day.) Two to five percent of hospital admissions are for iatrogenic disease; 18 percent of hospitalized patients develop drug reactions; at least three billion dollars is the annual cost of adverse drug reactions; and at least 1.5 million therapeutic drug mis-adventures occur each year, which is twice the number of persons treated for cancer.[212] Fatality rates from complications arising from coronary arteriography range from one to 80 per 1000.[213] Use of oral contraceptives significantly increases the risk of mycardial infarction.[214] Exposure to diethylstilbestrol (DES) definitely increases the risk of unfavorable pregnancy outcomes, and of benign vaginal and cervical changes.[215] A definite increased risk of Guillain-Barre syndrome occurred in 1976, resulting from the swine-influenza vaccine.[216] Radiation therapy is a significant cause of cancer.[217]

In general, since few of the adverse reactions shown under categories **1, 2, 6, 7, 9,** and **10** above are counted or recognized for what they are, we have no clear idea of the size of the problem of iatrogenicity. Given the tremendous and mounting size of the negative aspects of medical therapy, Illich has speculated on the declining marginal gains or increasing marginal losses from ever-more complicated and more widespread use of "scientific" medical interventions.[218]

All of us are going to have to deal with such complex issues as withholding oxygen and risking premature newborn lives, in order to avoid blindness caused by use of oxygen required to bring prematures through to an otherwise apparently normal, if visually impaired, life.[219]

In presenting the four areas of evidence about the factors that affect health, we have scanned a mountain of data, almost all of which is consistent with the general systems paradigm. That is, good health of individuals is assured by harmonious functioning and relationships among all levels of systems in the *homo sapiens* hierarchy. It requires a degree of equity, justice, and caring that we are very far from attaining. Ill-health represents perturbations and inharmonious relationships of the various systems levels. The massive ill-effects of supra-systems' perturbations on large numbers of individuals, the complex interrelationships of perturbations at one or more systems levels, and the complex outcomes of intended perturbations (e.g., therapy directed at any level of system), all speak to the utility of the general systems view of good and bad health.

REFERENCES

1. R. Dubos, *Mirage of Health,* New York, Harper, 1959. T. McKeown and C.R. Lowe, *An Introduction to Social Medicine,* Philadelphia, F. A. Davis and Company, 1966, Chapter 1. T. McKeown, *The Role of Medicine,* New Jersey, Princeton University Press, 1979.

2. W. Winkelstein, Jr., "Epidemiological Considerations Underlying the Allocation of Health and Disease Care Resources," *International Journal of Epidemiology,* 1972, 1:1, 69-74.

3. I. T. T. Higgins, "The Epidemiology of Chronic Respiratory Diseases," *Preventive Medicine,* 1973, 2, 14-33.

4. J. Powles, "The Medicine of Industrial Man," *The Ecologist,* 1972, 2:10, 198-204.

5. J. F. Fries and L. M. Crapo, *Vitality and Aging,* San Francisco, W. H. Freeman, 1981, 59-77. *World Development Report,* Washington, D.C., World Bank, August 1981, 175.

6. C. Bezold, *The Future of Pharmaceuticals,* New York, John Wiley and Sons, 1981.

7. J. F. Fries and L. M. Crapo, ibid. No. 5.

8. J. W. Ratcliffe, "U.S. Energy Policy and the Health Education Profession: Two Futures," paper prepared for presentation at the annual meeting of the Society for Public Health Education, Los Angeles, California, October 30, 1981. B. Lown, et al., "The Nuclear Arms Race and the Physician," *New*

England Journal of Medicine, 1981, (19 March), 304, 726-729. S. A. Fetter and K. Tsipis, "Catastrophic Releases of Radioactivity," *Scientific American,* 1981 (April), 244:4, 41-47. E. J. Steinglass, The Invisible Death (Part I): The First Casualty at T.M.I., *The Nation,* 1981, (28 February), 232:8, 225, 240-244. E. J. Steinglass, The Invisible Death (Part II): The Lethal Path of T.M.I. Fallout, *The Nation,* 1981, (7 March), 232:9, 267-269, 272-273. J. W. Ratcliffe, "Institute for Applied Research in Peace and Global Security: A Proposal," draft copy, School of Public Health, University of California, Berkeley, 1981, (18 September).

9. R. Cooper, "Blacks and Hypertension," *Urban Health,* 1975, 4:6, 9. R. Cooper, et al., "Racism, Society and Disease: An Exploration of the Social and Biological Mechanism of Differential Mortality," *International Journal of Health Services,* 1981, 11:3, 389-414. *Assessment of Technologies for Determining Cancer Risks from the Environment,* Office of Technology Assessment, Congress of the United States, June, 1981. *Health United States 1978,* US DHEW Publication No. (PHS) 78-1232, December 1978. *Health United States 1979,* US DHEW Publication No. (PHS) 80-1232, 1980. A. Kagan, "Epidemiology and Society, Stress and Disease," in L. Levi, *Society, Stress and Disease,* London: Oxford University Press, 1971, Volume 1, Chapter 5. T. W. Oakes and S. L. Syme, "Social Factors in Newly Discovered Elevated Blood Pressure," *Journal of Health and Social Behavior,* 1973, 14, 198-204. L. M. Verbrugge, "Sex Differentials in Health," *Public Health Reports,* Sept-Oct 1982, 97:5, 417-436.

10. J. Eyer, "Introduction to the Theme: The Economy, Medicine, and Health," *International Journal of Health Services,* 1977, 7:1, 3-6.

11. E. Cassell and D. Lebowitz, "Causality in the Environment and Health," *Perspectives in Biology and Medicine,* Spring, 1976, 19:3, 338-343.

12. E. S. Rogers and H. B. Messinger, "Human Ecology: Toward a Holistic Method," *Milbank Memorial Quarterly,* XIV:1, Part I, January 1967, 25-42.

13. S. L. Syme and L. F. Berkman, "Social Class, Susceptibility and Sickness," *American Journal of Epidemiology,* 1976, 104:1, 1-8. S. L. Syme and C. P. Torfs, "Epidemiologic Research in Hypertension: A Critical Appraisal," *Journal of Human Stress,* March 1978, 4:1, 43-48. S. L. Syme, M. M. Hyman, and P.E. Enterline, "Cultural Mobility and the Occurrence of Coronary Heart Disease," *Journal of Health and Human Behavior,* Winter, 1965, 6, 178-189. S. L. Syme, "Life Style Intervention in Clinic-Based Trials," *American Journal of Epidemiology,* 1978, 108:2, 87-91. R. G. Robinson, "Structural Conditions as a Basis for Understanding the Health of Population: Perspective on Policy Options and Strategies," paper presented at the Annual Conference of the African Heritage Studies Association and the National Conference of Black Political Scientists, Baltimore, Maryland, April 16-18, 1981.

14. J. W. Ratcliffe, "Notions of Validity in Qualitative Research Methodology," paper prepared for presentation of the Study Group Session Grounded Theory and Qualitative Methods organized by the Committee on Health Services Research (Medical Care Section), American Public Health Association, Annual Convention, Detroit, Michigan, October, 1980. P. Schwartz and J. Ogilvy, "The Emergent Paradigm: Changing Patterns of Thought and Belief," Analytical Report, No. 7, Values and Lifestyles Program, April, 1979.

15. *Health of the Disadvantaged: Chartbook,* US DHEW, PHS, HRA, September, 1977. D. B. Dutton, "Children's Health Care: The Myth of Equal

Access," in *Better Health for our Children: A National Strategy,* DHHS, PHS Pub. No. 79-55071, 1981, 357-440.

16. *Health U.S.A., 1978,* ibid, No. 9. *Health U.S.A., 1979,* ibid, No. 9. H. M. Brenner, "Health Costs and Benefits of Economic Policy," *International Journal of Health Services,* 1977, 7:4, 581-623. C. A. Laurell, et al., "Disease and Rural Development: A Sociological Analysis of Morbidity in Two Mexican Villages," *International Journal of Health Services,* 1977, 7:3, 401-423. A. Antonovsky and I. K. Zola (Eds.), *Poverty and Health,* Harvard University Press, 1969. D. Mechanic, "Social Justice," in R. M. Battistella and T. G. Rundall (Eds.), *Health Care Policy in a Changing Environment,* Berkeley, McCutchan Publishing Company, 1978, 253-273. J. R. Hochstim, et al., "Poverty Area Under the Microscope," *American Journal of Public Health,* October, 1968, 58:10, 1815-1827. E. M. Kitagawa and P. M. Hauser, *Differential Mortality in the United States,* Cambridge, Massachusetts, Harvard University Press, 1973. J. W. Ratcliffe, *Population Control Versus Social Justice: Political Economy of Population Policy.* New York, Monthly Review Press, Chapter 3, (in press).

17. S. L. Syme and L. F. Berkman, ibid, No. 13.

18. J. R. Hochstim, et al., "Poverty Area Under the Microscope," *American Journal of Public Health,* October, 1968, 58:10, 1815-1827.

19. B. Starfield, "Stability and Change: Another View," *American Journal of Public Health,* March 1981, 31:3, 301-302.

20. J. R. Hochstim, D. A. Athanasapoulus, and J. H. Larkens, "Poverty Area Under the Microscope," *American Journal of Public Health,* October, 1968, 58:10, 1815-1827. N. A. Holtzman, "Prevention: Rhetoric and Reality," *International Journal of Health Services,* 1979, 9:1, 25-36.

21. M. Fried, "Social Differences in Mental Health," in John Kosa, et al. (Eds.), *Poverty and Health,* Cambridge, Harvard University Press, 1969.

22. National Advisory Council on Economic Opportunity, *The American Promise: Equal Justice and Economic Opportunity,* (Final Report), September, 1981.

23. *Health U.S.A. 1979,* ibid, No. 9.

24. Ibid, No. 2.

25. M. H. Rudov and N. Santangelo, "Health Status of Minorities and Low Income Groups," US DHEW, PHS, (HRA) 79-627, 1979.

26. Technology Assessment, ibid, No. 9.

27. Ibid, No. 25.

28. R. Cooper, ibid., No. 9.

29. V. L. Ernster, et al., "Prostatic Cancer: Mortality and Incidence Rates by Race and Social Class," *American Journal of Epidemiology,* 1978, 107:4, 311-320.

30. Technology Assessment, ibid, No. 9.

31. W. E. Morton and G. F. Starr, "Epidemiologic Clues to the Cause of Melanoma," *The Western Journal of Medicine,* October, 1979, 131, 263-269.

32. *Health U.S.A. 1978,* ibid., No. 9. *Health U.S.A. 1979,* ibid, No. 9. T. A. DeRouen, "The Recent Decline in Heart Disease Mortality and Factors Related to It," *Washington Public Health,* Winter, 1981, 2:2, 5-8.

33. L. Pratt, "The Relationship of Socio-Economic Status to Health," *American Journal of Public Health,* 1971, 61:2, 281-91.

34. Ibid, No. 25.

35. S. L. Syme and L. F. Berkman, ibid, No. 13. S. A. James and D. G. Kleinbaum, "Socioecologic Stress and Hypertension Related Mortality Rates in North Carolina," *American Journal of Public Health,* April, 1976, 66:4, 354-358. H. A. Tyller and S. A. James, "Blood Pressure and Skin Color," *American Journal of Public Health,* December 1978, 68:12, 1170-1172. R. F. Gillum, "Pathophysiology of Hypertension in Blacks and Whites: A Review of the Basis of Racial Blood Differences," *Hypertension,* 1979, 1:5, 468-475. A. M. Ostfeld and D. A. D'Atri, "Rapid Sociocultural Change and High Blood Pressure," *Adv. Psychosomatic Medicine,* 1977, 9, 20-37. S. L. Syme, "Drug Treatment in Mild Hypertension: Social and Psychological Considerations," *Annals New York Academy of Science,* 1978, 99-106. J. Eyer, "Hypertension as a Disease of Modern Society," *International Journal of Health Services,* 1975, 5:4, 539-558.

36. A. Apostolides, et al., "High Blood Pressure: Its Care and Consequences in Urban Centres," *International Journal of Epidemiology,* 1974, 3:2, 105-118. D. Harris, et al., "The Child Adolescent Blood Pressure Study," *American Journal of Public Health,* December, 1981, 71:12, 1342-1349. F. J. DeCastro, et al., "Hypertension in Adolescents," *Clinical Pediatrics,* 1976, 15, 24-26.

37. S. L. Syme and L. F. Berkman, ibid, No. 13. S. L. Syme, "Drug Treatment in Mild Hypertension: Social and Psychological Considerations," *Annals New York Academy of Science,* 1978, 99-106.

38. J. Eyer, "Hypertension as a Disease of Modern Society," *International Journal of Health Services,* 1975, 5:4, 539-558.

39. G. E. Thomson and S. W. Lambert, "Hypertension: Implications of Comparisons Among Blacks and Whites," *Urban Health,* May 1980, 9:4, 31-33.

40. R. F. Gillum, "Pathophysiology of Hypertension in Blacks and Whites: A Review of the Basis of Racial Blood Differences," *Hypertension,* 1979, 1:5, 468-475. E. Harburg, et al., "Skin Color, Ethnicity, and Blood Pressure: Detroit Blacks," *American Journal of Public Health,* December, 1978, 68:12, 1177-1183.

41. Ibid, No. 25.

42. R. Cooper, ibid, No. 9.

43. R. Cooper, ibid, No. 9.

44. M. G. Marmot, et al., "Changing Social Class Distribution of Heart Disease," *British Medical Journal,* 1978, 2, 1109-1112. M. G. Marmot, et al., "Employment Grade and Coronary Heart Disease in British Civil Servants," *Journal of Epidemiology and Community Health,* December, 1978, 32:4, 244-249.

45. Ibid, No. 25.

46. J. Chapman and A. Coulson, "Community Diagnosis: An Analysis of Health and Disease in a Metropolitan Area," *International Journal of Epidemiology,* 1972, 1:1, 75-81. H. C. Chase (Ed.), "A Study of Risks, Medical Care and Infant Mortality," *American Journal of Public Health,* September, 1974, Supplement to Volume 63, R. Lewis, M. Charles, K. M. Patwary, "Relationships Between Birthweight and Selected Social Environmental and Medical Care Factors," *American Journal of Public Health,* 1963, 63:11, 973-81.

47. *Health U.S.A. 1978,* ibid, No. 9. *Health U.S.A. 1979,* ibid, No. 9.

48. *World Development Report,* Washington, D.C., World Bank, August, 1981, 175.

49. *Health U.S.A. 1979,* ibid, No. 9.

50. National Advisory Council on Economic Opportunity, *The American Promise: Equal Justice and Economic Opportunity,* (Final Report), September 1981. H. M. Brenner, "Fetal, Infant and Maternal Mortality During Periods of Economic Instability," *International Journal of Health Services,* Spring, 1973, 3:2, 145-159.

51. E. A. Krause, *Power and Illness: The Political Sociology of Health and Medical Care,* New York, Elsevier North-Holland, Inc., 1979.

52. D. Mechanic, *Medical Sociology,* New York, The Free Press, 1968, Chapter 7.

53. M. Behar, "A Deadly Combination, Malnutrition and Infectious Disease," *World Health,* WHO, Geneva, 1974, February-March, 28-33. J. M. Bengoa, "The Problem of Malnutrition," *WHO Chronicle,* 1974, 28, 3-7. J. M. Bengoa, "Hunger and Malnutrition," *World Health,* WHO, February-March, 1974. N. S. Scrimshaw, et al., "Nutrition and Infection Field Studies: Guatemalan Villages, 1959-64," *Archives of Environmental Health,* 1968, 16, 223-234. D. Calloway and C. Wood, "Nutrition as a Basic Need," Department of Nutritional Sciences, University of California, Berkeley, Nov. 1978, Mimeo.

54. S. L. Syme and L. F. Berkman, ibid, No. 13. H. Behn, "Demographic Growth and Health Needs in Latin America," *International Journal of Health Services,* 1979, 9:1, 77-85. USDHEW, "Changes in Population Structure," in R.M. Battistella and T. G. Rundall (Eds.), *Health Care Policy in a Changing Environment,* Berkeley: McCutchan Publishing Co., 1978, 88-119.

55. N. S. Scrimshaw and J. E. Gordon (Eds.), *Malnutrition, Learning and Behavior,* Cambridge: The MIT Press, 1968. J. Tizard, "Can the Brain Catch Up After Childhood Malnutrition," *World Health,* WHO, Geneva, 1974, February-March, 10-14. *WHO Chronicle, "Malnutrition and Mental Development,"* 1974, 28, 95-102.

56. R. Karp, et al., "Effects of Rise in Food Costs on Hemoglobin Concentrations of Early School-Age Children, 1972-75," *Public Health Reports,* 1978, September-October, 93:5, 456-459. S. Reutlinger and M. Selousky, "An Overview of Malnutrition and Poverty: Magnitude and Policy Options," *World Bank Staff Occasional Papers,* No. 23, The World Bank, 1976.

57. S. V. Kosl, "Effects of Residential Environment on Health and Behavior: A Review," a report written under contract CPE-R-69-30, to the Bureau of Community Environmental Management, HSMHA, PHS, DHEW, March, 1972. J. Kosa, A. Antonovsky, I. K. Zola, *Poverty and Health,* Cambridge, Harvard University Press, 1969.

58. J. Mann, "Dying Babies: America and the Third World," *Washington Post,* May 22, 1981.

59. J. M. Bengoa, "Hunger and Malnutrition," *World Health,* WHO, February-March, 1974. H. Behn, "Democratic Growth and Health Needs in Latin America," *International Journal of Health Services,* 1979, 9:1, 77-85. S. Reutlinger and M. Selousky, "An Overview of Malnutrition and Poverty: Magnitude and Policy Options," *World Bank Staff Occasional Papers,* No. 23, The World Bank, 1976. J. W. Ratcliffe, "Population Control Versus Social Reorganization: The Emergent Paradigm," *International Journal of Health Services,* 1978, 8:3, 559-568. B. Moss, *Population Target: The Political Economy of Population Control in Latin America,* Charters Publishing Co., Brampton, Ontario, Canada, 1976.

60. R. Cooper, ibid, No. 9.

61. J. Eyer, "Prosperity as a Cause of Death," *International Journal of Health Services,* 1977, 7:1, 125-150.

62. A. Antonovsky, "Social Class, Life Expectancy and Overall Mortality," *Milbank Memorial Fund Quarterly,* 1967, 45:1, 37-75. C. Kadushin, "Social Class and the Experience of Ill Health," *Sociological Inquiry,* 1964 (Winter), 34:1, 67-80. The World Bank, *The Assault on World Poverty: Problems of Rural Development, Education, and Health,* Baltimore, The Johns Hopkins University Press, 1975.

63. C. A. Laurell, ibid, No. 16.

64. R. G. Robinson, ibid, No. 13.

65. M. Turshen, "The Impact of Colonialism on Health Services in Tanzania," *International Journal of Health Services,* 1977, 7:1, 7-35. J. H. Geiger, "Community Control — or Community Conflict," *National Tuberculosis and Respiratory Disease Bulletin,* 1969, 55:10, 5-11. B. Moss, *Population Target: The Political Economy of Population Control in Latin America.* Charters Publishing Co., Brampton, Ontario, Canada, 1976. L. Doyal, *The Political Economy of Health,* South End Press, Boston, 1981, Ch. 3.

66. J. Ratcliffe, "Social Justice and the Demographic Transition: Lessons from India's Kerala State," *International Journal of Health Services,* 1978, 8:1, 123-144. E. S. Guttmacher and R. Danielson, "Changes in Cuban Health Care: An Argument Against Technological Pessimism," *International Journal of Health Services,* 1977, 7:3, 483-500. G. Salimono and P. Hakim, "Nutrition and National Development: The Case of Chile," *International Journal of Health Services,* 1979, 9:3, 495-510. D. Fetherston, "How Costa Rica Developed Its Model System of Health Care," *San Francisco Chronicle,* December 23, 1981.

67. J. W. Ratcliffe, ibid, No. 8. National Advisory Council on Economic Opportunity, *The American Promise: Equal Justice and Economic Opportunity,* (Final Report), September 1981. H. M. Brenner, "Fetal, Infant and Maternal Mortality During Periods of Economic Instability," *International Journal of Health Services,* Spring 1973, 3:2, 145-159. H. M. Brenner, *Mental Illness and*

the Economy, Cambridge, Harvard University Press, 1973. H. M. Brenner, "Economic Changes and Heart Disease Mortality," *American Journal of Public Health,* 1971, 61:3, 606-611. H. M. Brenner, "Trends in Alcohol Consumption and Associated Illnesses: Some Effects of Economic Changes," *American Journal of Public Health,* 1975, 65:12, 1279-1292. H. M. Brenner, Health Costs and Benefits of Economic Policy," *International Journal of Health Services,* 1977, 7:4, 581-623. H. M. Brenner, "Mortality and the National Economy: A Review and the Experience of England and Wales, 1936-1976," *Lancet,* September 15, 1979, 11:8142, 568-573. V. Lin, "Health and the Economy: Is Unemployment a Killer Disease?" a technical assistance memo, Western Center for Health Planning, November 18, 1980. A. R. Bunn, "Ischaemic Heart Disease Mortality and the Business Cycle in Australia," *American Journal of Public Health,* 1979 (August), 69:8, 772, 781. "Economy Has Direct Health Effects," *The Nation's Health,* 1977 (January). H. M. Brenner, "Cardiovascular Renal Disease Mortality and Economic Instability in the United States," paper given at annual meeting, APHA, San Francisco, November 8, 1973.

68. S. V. Kasl and S. Cobb, "Blood Pressure Changes of Men Undergoing Job Loss: A Preliminary Report," *Psychosomatic Medicine,* 1970, XXXII:I, 19-38.

69. A. Slote, *Termination: The Closing of Baker Plant,* Indianapolis, The Bobbs-Merrill Co., 1969.

70. J. Eyer, "Prosperity as a Cause of Death," *International Journal of Health Services,* 1977, 7:1, 125-150. J. Eyer, "Does Unemployment Cause the Death Rate Peak in Each Business Cycle? A Multifactor Model of Death Rate Changes," *International Journal of Health Services,* 1977, 7:4, 625-662. J. Eyer, "Review of Mental Illness and the Economy," *International Journal of Health Services,* 1976, 6:1, 239-248.

71. E. M. Kitagawa and P. M. Hauser, *Differential Mortality in the United States,* Cambridge, Massachusetts, Harvard University Press, 1973. "High Association is Found Between Education and Health," *The Nation's Health,* October, 1981.

72. Ibid, No. 25. J. Kosa, A. Antonovsky, and I. K. Zola, *Poverty and Health,* Cambridge, Harvard University Press, 1969. E. M. Kitagawa, "Social and Economic Differentials in Mortality in the United States, 1960," Presented at session on socio-economic differentials in mortality, General Assembly and Conference of International Union of Scientific Study of Population, London, September 3-11, 1969. E. M. Kitagawa and P. M. Hauser, *Differential Mortality in the United States,* Cambridge, Massachusetts, Harvard University Press, 1973. R. Cooper, ibid, No. 9. R. G. Robinson, ibid, No. 13. A. B. Goodman, "Re: Determining Social Class Differences in Illness Rates for Blacks and Whites," *American Journal of Epidemiology,* 1979, 109:3, 376-377. V. L. Ernster, "The First Author Replies," *American Journal of Epidemiology,* 1979, 109:3, 377-378.

73. A. B. Hollingshead and F. C. Redlich, *Social Class and Mental Illness: A Community Study,* New York, John Wiley and Sons, Inc., 1969, 387-397. A. B. Hollingshead, *Elmtown's Youth: The Impact of Social Classes on Adolescents,* New York, John Wiley and Sons, Inc., 1949. L. W. Warner, *Readings of Social Stratification,* Prentice-Hall, 1970, 228-257.

74. R. Centers, "Social Class, Occupation and Imputed Belief," *The American Journal of Sociology,* 1953 (May) LXIII:6, 543-555.

75. R. Fein, "An Economic and Social Profile of the Negro American," in *The Negro American,* Talcott Parsons and Kenneth B. Clark (Eds.), Boston, Beacon Press, 1966, 102-133. A. Billingsley, *Black Families in White America,* Prentice-Hall, Inc., 1968. D. K. Newman, et al., *Protest Politics and Prosperity: Black Americans and White Institutions,* New York, Pantheon Books, 1978.

76. R. Cooper, ibid, No. 9. R. G. Robinson, ibid, No. 13. A. B. Goodman, ibid, No. 72.

77. *Health U.S.A. 1978,* ibid, No. 9. E. A. Krause, *Power and Illness: The Political Sociology of Health and Medical Care,* Elsevier North-Holland, Inc., 1979.

78. L. V. Cralley (Ed.), *Industrial Environmental Health,* New York, Academic Press, 1972. M. Key, *Occupational Diseases: A Guide to Their Recognition,* USDHEW (N10SH) Publication No. 77-181, 1977. J. M. Stellman and S. Daum, *Work is Dangerous to Your Health,* New York, Vintage Books, 1973.

79. D. M. Berman, "Death on the Job: Occupational Health and Safety Struggles in the United States," *Monthly Review Press,* 1978.

80. *Health U.S.A. 1979,* ibid, No. 9.

81. C. D. McClure, "Public Health Concerns in the Exposure of Grape Pickers to High Pesticide Residues in Madera County, California, September 1976," *Public Health Reports,* 1978 (September-October) 93:5, 421-425.

82. Technology Assessment, ibid, No. 9. *Health U.S.A. 1979,* ibid, No. 9. R. J. Pasick, "Protection from Environmental Health Hazards Through Health Education and Health Planning," paper presented at the American Public Health Association Annual Conference, Los Angeles, California, October 17, 1978.

83. B. J. Castleman and M. J. Vera Vera, "Impending Proliferation of Asbestos," *International Journal of Health Services,* 1980, 10:3, 389-403.

84. *Health U.S.A. 1978,* ibid, No. 9.

85. Technology Assessment, ibid, No. 9.

86. W. E. Morton and G. F. Starr, "Epidemiologic Clues to the Cause of Melanoma," *The Western Journal of Medicine,* October, 1979, 131, 263-269.

87. R. Cooper, ibid, No. 9.

88. R. Cooper, ibid, No. 9.

89. E. A. Krause, ibid, No. 51. M. Davis, "The Impact of Workplace Health and Safety of Black Workers: Assessment and Prognosis," paper presented at the Annual American Industrial Hygiene Conference, Houston, Texas, May 21, 1980.

90. D. Baker, "The Use and Health Consequences of Shift Work," *International Journal of Health Services,* 1980, 10:3, 405-420.

91. A. Lebowitz, "Overview: The Health of Working Women," in *Women, Work, and Health: Challenges to Corporate Policy,* Springer-Verlag New York, Inc.,

1980. I. Waldron, "Employment and Women's Health: An Analysis of Causal Relationships," *International Journal of Health Services,* 1980, 10:3, 435-454.

92. A. Lebowitz, ibid, No. 91. N. J. Sokoloff, "Women's Work, Women's Health: Review and Analysis," *International Journal of Health Services,* 1980, 10:3.

93. J. M. Stellman, "The Biology of Toxic Effects in Reproductive Outcomes," in *Women, Work, and Health: Challenges to Corporate Policy,* Springer-Verlag New York, Inc., 1980.

94. D. M. Berman, "Death on the Job: Occupational Health and Safety Struggles in the United States," *Monthly Review Press,* 1978.

95. R. Crawford, "Individual Responsibility and Health Politics," in P. Conrad and R. Kein (Eds.), *Sociology of Health and Illness,* New York, St. Martin's Press, Inc., 1981, 468-481.

96. R. E. Mitchell, "Some Social Implications of High Density Housing," *American Sociological Review,* 1971 (February) 30, 18-29.

97. S. V. Kasl and E. Harburg, "Mental Health and the Urban Environment: Some Doubts and Second Thoughts," *Journal of Health and Social Behavior,* 1975 (September), 16:3, 268-282.

98. L. Levy and A. N. Herzog, "Effects of Population Density and Crowding on Health and Social Adaptation," *Netherlands Journal of Health and Social Behavior,* 1974, 15:3, 228-240.

99. L. Schweitzer and Wen-Huey Su, "Population Density and the Rate of Mental Illness," *American Journal of Public Health,* 1977, 67:12, 1165-1172.

100. A. M. Ostfeld and D. A. D'Atri, "Rapid Sociocultural Change and High Blood Pressure," *Adv. Psychosomatic Medicine,* 1977, 9, 20-37. D. A. D'Atri and A. M. Ostfeld, "Crowding: Its Effects on the Elevation of Blood Pressure in a Prison Setting," *Preventive Medicine,* 1975, 4, 550-566.

101. D. M. Wilner, "Sociocultural Factors of Residential Space," a report written under contract #PH 86-68-154 of the Bureau of Community Environmental Management, HSM, PHS, DHEW, 1970.

102. J. J. Wesolowski, et al., "Lead in the Blood of California Children," *The Western Journal of Medicine,* 1977 (September), 127, 271-273.

103. I. DeGroot, et al., "Human Health and Spatial Environment: An Epidemiological Assessment," a report written under contract PH 86-68-154 of the Bureau of Community Environmental Management, HSMHA, PHS, DHEW, undated.

104. S. V. Kasl, "Effects of Residential Environment on Health and Behavior—A Review," a report written under contract CPE-R-69-30 to the Bureau of Community Environmental Management, HSMHA, PHS, DHEW, March 1972.

105. Technology Assessment, ibid, No. 9.

106. W. Winkelstein, Jr., ibid, No. 2.

107. R. S. Chapman, et al., "Chronic Respiratory Disease," *Archives of Envionmental Health,* 1973 (September) 27, 138-142. C. M. Shy, et al., "Air Pollution

Effects on Ventilatory Function of U.S. School Children," *Archives of Environmental Health,* 1973, 17, 124-133.

108. R. J. Pasick, ibid, No. 82. L. Levy and A. N. Herzog, ibid, No. 98.

109. G. W. Comstock, et al., "Respiratory Findings and Urban Living," *Archives of Environmental Health,* 1973 (September) 27, 143-154.

110. R. W. Bueckly, et al., "SO_2 Levels and Perturbations in Mortality," *Archives of Environmental Health,* 1973, 27, 134-137.

111. B. W. Carnow and P. Meier, "Air Pollution and Pulmonary Cancer," *Archives of Environmental Health,* 1973, 27, 207-218.

112. Technology Assessment, ibid, No. 9. S. L. Syme and L. F. Berkman, ibid, No. 13.

113. Technology Assessment, ibid, No. 9.

114. R. J. Caprio, H. L. Margulies, and M. M. Joselow, "Exhaust Lead Seen as Hazard," as reported in *American Medical News,* 1974 (April 15), 27.

115. B. Brenner, I. Cisin, C. Newcomb, "Drinking Practices and Accidental Injuries," paper presented at the session on Alcohol Use and Accidents, Society for Study of Social Problems, Miami Beach, Florida, 1966 (August 26). Arthur D. Little, Inc., *The State of the Art of Traffic Safety—Summary Report,* Cambridge, 1966 (June) C-62270. *Social Forces and the Nation's Health,* HSMHA, PHS, USDHEW, 1968 (May). "Traffic Control and Roadway Elements: Their Relationship to Highway Safety," *Traffic Safety,* 1964, 8:3, 76. J. A. Waller, "The Role of Alcohol in Collisions Involving Trucks," *Archives of Environmental Health,* 1970, 20, 254-258. J. A. Waller, "Truth, Traps and Tactics Concerning Alcohol, Other Drugs and Highway Safety," *California Medicine,* 1972, 116, 10-15.

116. J. R. Goldsmith and E. Jonsson, "Health Effects of Community Noise," *American Journal of Public Health,* 1973 (September) 63:9, 782-793. S. Cohen and N. Weinstein, "Nonauditory Effects of Noise on Behavior and Health," *Journal of Social Issues,* 1981, 37:1, 36-70. S. Cohen, "Aircraft Noise and Children: Longitudinal and Cross-Sectional Evidence on Adaptation to Noise and the Effectiveness of Noise Abatement," *Journal of Personality and Social Psychology,* 1981, 40:2, 331-345. S. Cohen, et al., "Physiological, Motivational, and Cognitive Effects of Aircraft Noise on Children," *American Psychologist,* 1980 (March) 35:3, 231-243. S. Cohen, "Sound Effects on Behavior," *Psychology Today,* 1981 (October) 15:10, 38-49.

117. L. E. Hinkle, Jr., "The Concept of Stress in the Biological and Social Sciences," *Science, Medicine and Man,* 1973, 1, 31-48. R. S. Lazarus, "The Concepts of Stress and Disease," in L. Levi (Ed.), *Society, Stress and Disease,* London, Oxford University Press, 1971, 1, Chapter 7. L. Levi, *Society, Stress and Disease,* London, Oxford University Press, 1971, Volume 1, 1976, Volume 2.

118. S. Cohen and N. Weinstein, "Nonauditory Effects of Noise on Behavior and Health," *Journal of Social Issues,* 1981, 37:1, 36-70.

119. S. V. Kasl and E. Harburg, ibid, No. 97. J. Cassel and L. Waller, "The Relation of the Urban Environment to Health: Towards a Conceptual Frame and a Research Strategy," a report written under contract CPE R-69-30 of the Bureau of Community Environmental Management, HSMHA, PHS, DHEW, undated.

120. S. L. Syme and C. P. Torfs, "Epidemiologic Research in Hypertension: A Critical Appraisal," *Journal of Human Stress,* March, 1978, 4:1, 43-48. E. Harburg, et al., "Sociological Stressor Areas and Black-White Blood Pressure: Detroit," *Journal of Chronic Disease,* 1973, 26, 595-611. S. A. James and D. G. Kleinbaum, "Socioecologic Stress and Hypertension Related Mortality Rates in North Carolina," *American Journal of Public Health,* April, 1976, 66:4, 354-358. R. F. Gillum, "Pathophysiology of Hypertension in Blacks and Whites: A Review of the Basis of Racial Blood Differences," *Hypertension,* 1979, 1:5, 468-475. W. B. Neser, H. A. Tyroler, and J. C. Cassel, "Social Disorganization and Stroke Mortality in the Black Population of North Carolina," *American Journal of Epidemiology,* 1970 (August) 93:3, 166-175. A. Ruskin, O. W. Beard, and R. L. Schaffe, "Blast Hypertension: Elevated Arterial Pressures in the Victims of the Texas City Disaster," *American Journal of Medicine,* 1948, 4, 228-236. S. V. Kasl and S. Cobb, "Blood Pressure Changes of Men Undergoing Job Loss: A Preliminary Report," *Psychosomatic Medicine,* 1970, XXXII:I, 19-38.

121. E. Harburg, et al., "Socio-Ecological Stress, Suppressed Hostility, Skin Color, and Black-White Male Blood Pressure: Detroit," *Psychosomatic Medicine,* 1973 (July-August) 35:4, 276-296. E. Harburg, et al., "Skin Color, Ethnicity, and Blood Pressure: Detroit Blacks," *American Journal of Public Health,* December, 1978, 68:12, 1177-1183.

122. H. A. Tyroler and S. A. James, "Blood Pressure and Skin Color," *American Journal of Public Health,* December 1978, 68:12, 1170-1172. J. Keil, H. Tyroler, and E. Boyle, "Hypertension Effects of Social Class and Racial Admixture: The Results of a Cohort Study in the Black Population of Charleston, S.C.," *American Journal of Public Health,* 1977, 67, 634-639.

123. S. L. Syme, M. M. Hyman, and P. E. Enterline, "Cultural Mobility and the Occurrence of Coronary Heart Disease," *Journal of Health and Human Behavior,* Winter, 1965, 6, 178-189.

124. J. R. Bloom, "Social Support Systems and Cancer: A Conceptual View," in J. Cohen, J. Cullen, and R. Morten (Eds.), *Psychosocial Dimensions of Cancer: Some Research Issues,* New York, Rover Press, 1980. A. Antonovsky, *Health, Stress, and Coping,* San Francisco, Jossey Bass, 1979. M. Minkler, "Applications of Social Support Theory to Health Education: Implications for Work with the Elderly," *Health Education Quarterly,* 1981, 8:2, 147-165.

125. S. V. Kasl, ibid, No. 57.

126. A. Kagan, ibid, No. 9.

127. J. Cassel and L. Waller, ibid, No. 119.

128. H. Gans, *The Urban Villagers,* New York, Free Press, 1962, 281-305.

129. C. Killian, "Effect of Geriatric Transfers on Mortality Rates," *Social Work,* 1970 (January), 19-26.

130. M. Susser, "Widowhood: A Situational Life Stress or a Stressful Life Event?" *American Journal of Public Health,* 1981 (August), 71:8, 793-795. H. J. Thurlow, "General Susceptibility to Illness: A Selected Review," *The Canadian Medical Association Journal,* 1967 (December 2), 97, 1397-1404.

131. R. H. Rahe and J. Arthur, "Life Change and Illness Studies: Past History and Future Directions," *Journal of Human Stress,* 1978 (March) 4:1, 3;14. A. Slote, *Termination: The Closing of Baker Plant,* Indianapolis, The Bobbs-Merril Company, 1969.

132. J. Eyer, "Hypertension as a Disease of Modern Society," *International Journal of Health Services,* 1975, 5:4, 539-558. M. Frankenhaeuser, "Coping with Stress at Work," *International Journal of Health Services,* 1981, 11:4, 491-510.

133. Ibid, No. 22.

134. J. Garfield, "Alienated Labor, Stress, and Coronary Disease," *International Journal of Health Services,* 1980, 10:4, 551-561. S. V. Kasl, "The Effects of Stress and Other Psychosocial Factors in the Development of Coronary Heart Disease," *Washington Public Health,* 1981 (Winter) 2:2, 18-21.

135. P. Pancheri, et al., "Infarct as a Stress Agent: Life History and Personality Characteristics in Improved versus Not-Improved Patients After Severe Heart Attack," *Journal of Human Stress,* 1978 (March) 4:1, 16-22, 41.

136. T. H. Holmes and M. Masuda, "Psychosomatic Syndrome: When Mothers-in-Law or Other Disasters Visit, a Person Can Develop a Bad, Bad Cold, or Worse," *Psychology Today,* 1972 (April), 71-72, 106. T. H. Holmes and M. Masuda, "Life Changes and Illness Susceptibility," presented at a Symposium on Separation and Depression: Clinical and Research Aspects at the Annual Meeting of AAAS, Chicago, Illinois, December 26-20, 1970. T. H. Holmes and M. Masuda, *Life Changes and Illness: Susceptibility in Stressful Life Events,* New York, Wiley-Interscience, 1974.

137. R. H. Rahe and R. J. Arthur, "Life Change and Illness Studies: Past History and Future Directions," *Journal of Human Stress,* 1978 (March) 4:1, 3-14. J. G. Bruhn, "Effects of Chronic Illness on the Family," *The Journal of Family Practice,* 1977, 4:6, 1057-1060. L. E. Hinkle, Jr., "The Concept of Stress in the Biological and Social Sciences," *Science, Medicine and Man,* 1973, 1, 31-48.

138. J. H. Knowles, "The Responsibility of the Individual," in P. Conrad and R. Kein (Eds.), *The Sociology of Health and Illness,* New York, St. Martin's Press, 1981, 452-468. K. G. Bauer, *Improving the Chances for Health,* San Francisco, National Center for Health Education, 1981.

139. N. B. Belloc and L. Breslow, "Relationship of Physical Health Status and Health Practices," *Preventive Medicine,* 1972, 1:3, 409-421. N. B. Belloc, "Relationship of Health Practices and Mortality," *Preventive Medicine,* 1973, 2:1, 67-81.

140. S. L. Syme and C. P. Torfs, "Epidemiologic Research in Hypertension: A Critical Appraisal," *Journal of Human Stress,* March, 1978, 4:1, 43-48. M. G. Marmot, et al., "Changing Social Class Distribution of Heart Disease," *British Medical Journal,* 1978, 2, 1109-1112.

141. R. Cooper, "Rising Death Rates in the Soviet Union: The Impact of Coronary Heart Disease," *New England Journal of Medicine,* 1981 (21 May), 304:21, 1259-1265.

142. Technology Assessment, ibid, No. 9.

143. *Health U.S.A. 1979,* ibid, No. 9.

144. I. T. T. Higgins, "The Epidemiology of Chronic Respiratory Diseases," *Preventive Medicine,* 1973, 2, 14-33. L. Pederson, et al., "Change in Smoking Status Among School-Aged Youth: Impact of a Smoking Awareness Curriculum, Attitudes, Knowledge, and Environmental Factors," *American Journal of Public Health,* 1981 (December), 71-12, 1401-1404.

145. S. E. Holck, et al., "Lung Cancer Mortality and Smoking Habits: Mexican American Women," *American Journal of Public Health,* 1982 (January) 72:1, 38-42.

146. *Health U.S.A. 1978,* ibid, No. 9.

147. T. A. DeRouen, "The Recent Decline in Heart Disease Mortality and Factors Related to It," *Washington Public Health,* Winter, 1981, 2:2, 5-8. J. K. Kleinman, et al., "The Effects of Changes in Smoking Habits on Coronary Heart Disease Mortality," *American Journal of Public Health,* 1979 (August) 69:8, 795-802.

148. S. L. Syme and C. P. Torfs, ibid, No. 120. T. A. DeRouen, ibid, No. 147. A. M. Ostfeld and D. A. D'Atri, "Rapid Sociocultural Change and High Blood Pressure," *Adv. Psychosomatic Medicine,* 1977, 9, 20-37.

149. J. J. Polich, et al., "Childhood Obesity," *The Journal of Family Practice,* 1978, 7:4, 849-855.

150. Technology Assessment, ibid, No. 9.

151. S. Grundy, "Can Changes in the American Diet Reduce the Likelihood of Developing Coronary Heart Disease?" *Washington Public Health,* 1981 (Winter) 2:2, 13-17.

152. Ibid, No. 151.

153. B. Armstrong, A. J. Van Merwyk, and H. Coates, "Blood Pressure in Seventh Day Adventist Vegetarians," *American Journal of Epidemiology,* 1977, 105, 444-449. L. McEvoy and G. Land, "Life-Style and Death Patterns of the Missouri RLDS Church Members," *American Journal of Public Health,* December, 1981, 71:12, 1350-1356. R. L. Phillips, et al., "Coronary Heart Disease Mortality Among SDA with Differing Dietary Habits," *American Journal of Clinical Nutrition,* 1978, 31:Supplement 6191-6198. R. D. Harris, et al., "The Child-Adolescent Blood Pressure Study: Distribution of Blood Pressure Levels in Seventh-Day Adventist (SDA) and Non-SDA Children," *American Journal of Public Health,* December, 1981, 71:12, 1342-1349. J. Higginson, "A Hazardous Society? Individual versus Community Responsibility in Cancer Prevention," *American Journal of Public Health,* 1976 (April) 66:4, 359-366.

154. T. A. DeRouen, ibid, No. 147. M. G. Marmot, et al., ibid, No. 140.

155. J. H. Knowles, ibid, No. 138.

156. Technology Assessment, ibid, No. 9.

157. I. Colon, "Alcohol Availability and Cirrhosis Mortality Rates by Genes and Race," *American Journal of Public Health,* 1981 (December) 71:12, 1325-1328.

158. J. H. Knowles, ibid, No. 138.

159. R. D. Nashold and E. M. Noor, "Alcohol-Related Deaths in Wisconsin: The Impact of Alcohol on Mortality," *American Journal of Public Health,* 1981 (November) 71:11, 1237-1241. J. A. Waller, "The Role of Alcohol in Collisions Involving Trucks," *Archives of Environmental Health,* 1970, 20, 254-258. J. L. Waller, "Truth, Traps, and Tactics Concerning Alcohol, Other Drugs and Highway Safety," *California Medicine,* 1972, 116, 10-15.

160. V. Froelicher, "Can Exercise Prevent Coronary Heart Disease?" *Washington Public Health,* 1981 (Winter) 2:2, 9-12. S. M. Fox and J. S. Skinner, "Physical Activity and Cardiovascular Health," *American Journal of Cardiology,* 1964, 14:6, 731-745. *The Framingham Heart Study,* U.S. DHEW PHS Publication #1515, 1966.

161. N. B. Belloc and L. Breslow, ibid, No. 139. L. Pratt, "The Relationship of Socio-Economic Status to Health," *American Journal of Public Health,* 1971, 61:2, 281-291.

162. *Health U.S.A. 1979,* ibid, No. 9.

163. Ibid, No. 25.

164. Ibid, No. 25.

165. R. E. Baranow, "The American Woman: What are Her Chances Against Cancer in 1967?" *Journal of American Medical Association,* 1966 (26 December) 19873, 39-40.

166. Ibid, No. 25. "Women Ignoring Cancer Checks," *Health Resources,* 1974 (December) 2:4.

167. E. J. Schaefer and J. R. Hughes, "Socioeconomic Factors and Maternal and Child Health Care," *Medical Care,* 1976 (June) XIV:6, 535-543.

168. D. Fife, et al., "Relative Mortality of Unbelted Infant Passengers and Belted Non-Infant Passengers in Air Accidents with Survivors," *American Journal of Public Health,* 1981 (November) 71:11, 1242-1246.

169. J. R. Bloom, "Social Support Systems and Cancer: A Conceptual View," in J. Cohen, J. Cullen, and R. Morten (Eds.), *Psychosocial Dimensions of Cancer: Some Research Issues,* New York, Raven Press, 1980. W. A. Satariano and S. L. Syme, "Life Change and Disease: Coping with Change," revised version of paper presented to the Conference on Biology and Behavior of the Elderly, National Academy of Science, Woods Hole, Massachusetts, June 22-24, 1979. R. Hessler, et al., "Demographic Context, Social Interaction, and Perceived Health Status: Excedrin Headache #1," *Journal of Health and Social Behavior,* 1971 (September) 12, 191-199. J. R. Bloom, "The Effect of Social Support on Patient Adjustment After Breast Surgery," *Patient Counseling and Health Education,* 1978 (Fall) 1:2, 50-59. I. Illich, *Medical Nemesis: The Expropriation of Health,* London, Marion Boyars, 1975. B. Raphael, "Preventive Intervention with the Recently Bereaved," *Archives General Psychiatry,* 1977, 34, 1450-1454. M. Pilisuk and S. Parks, "Structural Dimensions of Social Support Groups," *Journal of Psychology,* 1980, 106, 157-177.

170. J. Powles, "The Medicine of Industrial Man," *The Ecologist,* 1972, 2:10, 24-36.

171. A. Kagan, ibid, No. 9.

172. A. Calin, "The Relationships Between Genetics and Environment in the Pathogenesis of Rheumatic Disease," *The Western Journal of Medicine,* 1979 (September) 131, 205-218.

173. A. G. Bearn and E. D. Kilbourne, "Genetic Determinants of Health and Disease," 29-46 in E. D. Kilbourne and W. G. Smithe (Eds.), *Human Ecology and Public Health,* Macmillan Company, London, 1969. V. A. McKusick, "Ethnic Distribution of Disease," *The Journal of Chronic*

Disease, 1967 (20 March), 115-118. V. A. McKusick, *Human Genetics,* Englewood Cliffs, Prentice Hall, 1969, 2nd Edition.

174. *WHO Chronicle,* "Pharmacogenetics—The Influence of Heredity on the Response to Drugs," 1974, 28, 25-31.

175. A. G. Bearn and E. D. Kilbourne, "Genetic Determinants of Health and Disease," 29-46 in E. D. Kilbourne and W. G. Smithe (Eds.), *Human Ecology and Public Health,* Macmillan Company, London, 1969.

176. N. A. Holtzman, "Prevention: Rhetoric and Reality," *International Journal of Health Services,* 1979, 9:1, 25-36. J. P. Newhouse and L. J. Friedlander, "The Relationship Between Medical Resources and Measures of Health: Some Additional Evidence," *The Journal of Human Resources,* 1980 (Spring) 15:2, 200-218. *Forward Plan for Health,* FY 1977-1981, Publication No. (05) 76-50024, USDHEW, 1975. M. Lalonde, *A New Perspective in the Health of Canadians,* Government of Canada, Ottawa, 1974. J. B. McKinlay and S. M. McKinlay, "The Questionable Contribution of Medical Measures to the Decline of Mortality in the United States in the Twentieth Century," *Milbank Memorial Fund Quarterly/Health and Society,* 1977 (Summer) 405-428. D. Mechanic, "Health and Illness in Technological Societies," *The Hastings Center Studies,* 1973, 6:3, 7-18. J. W. Ratcliffe, *Population Control versus Social Justice: Political Economy of Population Policy,* New York, Monthly Review Press, Chapter 3 (in press). J. Hadley, *More Medical Care, Better Health: An Economic Analysis of Mortality Rates,* Washington, D.C., The Urban Institute, 1981.

177. J. F. Fries and L. M. Crapo, *Vitality and Aging,* San Francisco, W. H. Freeman, 1981, 59-77.

178. A. L. Childs, "The Functions of Medical Care," *Public Health Reports,* 1975, 90:1, 10-14.

179. C. T. Stewart, Jr., "Allocation of Resources to Health," *The Journal of Human Resources,* 1971, 6:1, 103-22. J. W. Ratcliffe, *Population Control versus Social Justice: Political Economy of Population Policy,* New York, Monthly Review Press, Chapter 3 (in press).

180. The World Bank, *The Assault on World Poverty: Problems of Rural Development, Education, and Health,* Baltimore, The Johns Hopkins University Press, 1975.

181. R. Auster, I. Leveson, and D. Sarachek, "The Production of Health, An Exploratory Study," *The Journal of Human Resources,* 1969, 10:4, 411-436.

182. R. J. Haggerty, "The Boundaries of Health Care," *The Pharos,* 1972, 35:3, 106-111.

183. C. H. Goodrich, M. C. Olendzki, and G. S. Reader, *Welfare Medical Care,* Cambridge, Harvard University Press, 1970.

184. N. S. Scrimshaw, et al., "Nutrition and Infection Field Studies, Guatemalan Villages, 1959-64," *Archives of Environmental Health,* 1968, 16, 223-234.

185. W. McDermott, K. W. Deuschle, and C. R. Barnett, "Health Care Experiment at Many Farms," *Science,* 1972 (2 January) 175, 23-31.

186. J. H. Geiger, "Community Control—Or Community Conflict," *National Tuberculosis and Respiratory Disease Bulletin,* 1969, 55:10, 5-11. W. L.

Berggren, et al., "Reduction of Mortality in Rural Haiti Through a Primary Health Care Program," *The New England Journal of Medicine,* 1981 (28 May) 304:22, 1324-1330. B. S. Levy, "Reducing Neonatal Mortality Rates with Nurse Midwives," *American Journal of Obstetrics and Gynecology,* 1971, 109, 50-58.

187. J. A. H. Lee, S. L. Morrison and J. N. Marks, "Fatality from Three Common Surgical Conditions in Teaching and Non-Teaching Hospitals," *Lancet,* 1957, 785-790.

188. W. Silverman, "Medical Inflation," *Perspectives in Biology and Medicine,* Summer, 1980, 617-637. A. Donabedian, "The Quality of Medical Care: Methods for Assessing and Monitoring the Quality of Care for Research and for Quality Assurance Programs," in *Health U.S.A. 1978,* USDHEW, Publication No. (PHS) 78-1232, 1978 (December) 111-126.

189. E. Hemminki and A. Paakkulainen, "The Effects of Antibiotics on Mortality from Infectious Diseases in Sweden and Finland," *American Journal of Public Health,* 1976, 66:12, 1180-1184.

190. T. McKeown and C. R. Lowe, *An Introduction to Social Medicine,* Philadelphia, F. A. Davis Company, 1966. T. McKeown, *The Role of Medicine,* New Jersey, Princeton University Press, 1979.

191. H. G. Mather, et al., "Acute Myocardial Infarction: Home and Hospital Treatment," *British Medical Journal,* 1971, 3, 334-338.

192. J. I. Haft, "Stress Induced Platelet Clumps Tied to Infarct," as reported in the *Hospital Tribune,* 1974, 8:2, 5.

193. A. P. Hallstrom, "Medic I—Ten Years Experience," *Washington Public Health,* 1981 (March) 2:2, 27-28.

194. L. D. Fisher, "Evaluation of Survival with Coronary Bypass Surgery," *Washington Public Health,* 1981 (March) 2:2, 22-25.

195. R. Cooper, et al., "Improved Mortality Among U.S. Blacks 1968-78: The Role of Anti-Racist Struggle," *International Journal of Health Services,* 1981, 11:4, 511-522.

196. R. J. Havlik and M. Feinleib (Eds.), *Proceedings of the Conference on the Decline in Coronary Heart Disease Mortality,* USDHEW, NIH, Washington, D.C., Publication No. 79-1610, 1979. M. P. Stern, "The Recent Decline in Ischemic Heart Disease Mortality," *Ann. Intern. Med.,* 1979, 91, 630-640.

197. N. A. Holtzman, ibid, No. 176.

198. J. Newport, "Comparative Studies of Patterns of Maternity Care and Pregnancy Outcomes Among MediCal Mothers Receiving Care Under Different Arrangements for Financing and Delivery of Services," Medical Project Report #5, 1972 (November), School of Public Health, U.C.L.A., Los Angeles. B. S. Levy, et al., "Reducing Neonatal Mortality Rates with Nurse Midwives," *American Journal of Obstetrics and Gynecology,* 1971, 109, 50-58.

199. M. Tayback, et al., *Evaluation Studies on Maternal and Infant Care Project: Final Report,* University of Maryland, 1973.

200. The World Bank, *The Assault on World Poverty: Problems of Rural Development, Education, and Health,* Baltimore, The Johns Hopkins University Press, 1975.

201. I. Gordis, "Effectiveness of Comprehensive-Care Programs in Preventing Rheumatic Fever," *New England Journal of Medicine,* 1973, 289, 331-335.

202. N. A. Holtzman, ibid, No. 176. N. N. Morris, et al., "Shifting Age-Parity Distribution of Births and the Decreased Infant Mortality," *American Journal of Public Health,* 1975, 65, 359-362.

203. Community Nutrition Institute, *Weekly Report,* Washington, D.C., 1981 (March 5) XI:10.

204. H. C. Chase (Ed.), "A Study of Risks, Medical Care and Infant Mortality," *American Journal of Public Health,* September, 1974, Supplement to Volume 63. R. L. Williams, "Explaining a Health Care Paradox," *Policy Sciences,* 1975 (March) 6, 91-101. National Center for Health Statistics, "A Study of Infant Mortality from Linked Records by Age of Mother, Birth Order, and Other Variables," USDHEW, PHS, HRA, Vital and Health Statistics Series 20: No. 14, HEW Publications HRA 74-1851, 1973 (September).

205. R. Lewis, M. Charles, K. M. Patwary, "Relationships Between Birthweight and Selected Social Environmental and Medical Care Factors," *American Journal of Public Health,* 1963, 63:11, 973-981.

206. F. J. Ingelfinger, "Medicine: Meritorious or Meretricious," *Science,* 1978 (26 May) 200:4344, 942-946. W. Foege, quoted in *Hospital Week,* March 12, 1982: 18:2.

207. *Joint Newsletter,* California State Department of Health and State Office of Narcotics and Drug Abuse, 1974, 1:1, 3.

208. A. B. Bergman and S. J. Stamm, "The Morbidity of Cardiac Non-Disease in School Children," *The New England Journal of Medicine,* 1967, 276-18, 1008-1013. J. R. Bloom and S. Monterossa, "Hypertension Labeling and Sense of Well-Being," *American Journal of Public Health,* 1981 (November) 71:11, 1228-1236.

209. R. Nader, Testimony to the Senate Health Subcommittee as reported in the *San Francisco Chronicle,* December 19, 1973, page 14, column 1.

210. E. Hemminki, "Adverse Reactions to Antibiotic Drugs: The Present Scope of the Problem in Outpatient Care and Possibilities for Improvement," *International Journal of Health Services,* 1981, 11:2, 283-301.

211. University of California at San Francisco, "Drug Induced Lung Disease: The Price of Progress," Medical Staff Conference, *California Medicine,* 1973, 119, 48-55.

212. Ibid, No. 211. G. J. Caranasos, R. B. Stewart, and L. E. Cluff, "Drug Induced Illness Leading to Hospitalization," *Journal of American Medical Association,* 1974, 228:6, 713-717.

213. S. A. Schroeder, "The Complications of Coronary Arteriography: A Problem That Won't Go Away," *American Heart Journal,* 1980 (February) 99:2, 139-141.

214. D. Stone, et al., "Risk of Myocardial Infarction in Relation to Current and Discontinued Use of Oral Contraceptives," *The New England Journal of Medicine,* 1981 (20 August) 305:8, 420-424.

215. A. B. Barnes, "Fertility and Outcome of Pregnancy in Women Exposed in Utero to Diethylstilbestrol," *The New England Journal of Medicine,* 1980 (13 March) 302:11, 609-613. S. J. Robboy, et al., "Pathologic Findings in Young Women Enrolled in the National Cooperative Diethylstilbestrol Adenosis (DESAD) Project," *Obstetrics and Gynecology,* 1979 (March) 53:3, 309-317. P. C. O'Brian, et al., "Vaginal Epithelial Changes in Young Women Enrolled in the National Cooperative Diethylstilbestrol Adenosis (DESAD) Project," *Obstetrics and Gynecology,* 1979 (March) 53:3, 300-308.

216. E. S. Hurvity, et al., "Guillain-Barre Syndrome and the 1978-1979 Influenza Vaccine," *The New England Journal of Medicine,* 1981 (25 June) 304:26, 1557-1561.

217. F. S. Greenspan, "Thyroid Nodules and Thyroid Cancer," *The Western Journal of Medicine,* 1974, 121:5, 359-365.

218. I. Illich, *Medical Nemesis: The Expropriation of Health,* London, Marion Boyars, 1975.

219. W. K. Cross, "Scylla and Charybdis," as reported in the *Hospital Tribune,* 1974, 8:2, 7.

Chapter 4

EFFECTIVE HEALTH CARE: THE REQUIRED PROCESSES AND RELATIONSHIPS

My *Requirements for Effective Health Care* represent the results of a crude systems analysis (which we have just completed in **Chapters 2** and **3**) of "health as the outcome of interactions among the various systems levels in the *homo sapiens* hierarchy of natural systems." This has been filtered by my value hierarchy, which has, of course, been conditioned by my professional training in medicine and public health (see **Boxes B** and **D** in **Figure 1.1**, page **4**). Because my value base has not been made explicit up to this point, I spell it out now. Included are: 1) **widely-participative decision making**, i.e., democracy, 2) **maximal personal liberties**, under a framework of reasonable laws that do not permit significant infringement on the rights of others, 3) **equity of opportunity**, and 4) **equity of access** to such basic services as food, shelter, health care, and education, so that equity of opportunity becomes more than a slogan.

These two sets of forces that have shaped my thinking and behavior lead me to seek the goal of better health, as represented by improvements in all its 12 facets portrayed in **Figure 2.4** (page **22-3**).

Of course, my analytic processes are also guided by my beliefs about individual and organizational behavior. The extensive literature on behavior can be made, at the moment, to support almost any posture; I choose to take one that suggests that people generally will become more interested in the world around them and its effects on them by being given responsibility and authority as well as the opportunity for sharing in what is going on around them.[1] This does not guarantee that their responses will be to behave in a way that promotes their well-being, as I define it. But, under the forthcoming proposals, they at least will have had the opportunity to understand how they can help effect their own well-being and that of others; thus, they could presumably make more enlightened decisions accordingly.

Persons having other beliefs about human responses might emerge from their analyses about how to promote good health with different "requirements": persons holding different paradigms about the forces affecting health and the nature of well-being will probably emerge with other requirements. Persons holding different societal and professional values will surely also see the need for still other requirements that match their concepts. New experiences, of course, will provide new perceptions about health paradigms, new knowledge about human behavior, and new beliefs and new proposals for better health interventions.[2]

With these caveats in mind, I will assume, for the sake of developing this thesis, that we are together on my version of the contents of **Boxes A** through **D** in **Figure 1.1** (page **4**). We are now going to develop what it is that a "good" health care system must be prepared to offer if it is to meet the expectations already presented.

What I want to emphasize in this chapter are the attributes of health care that I think are of supreme importance. My service concerns can be organized into three major areas: 1) the **traditional care and cure** aspects of human services, 2) the **self-care** or **micro** activities, and 3) the **collective** or **macro** activities. All three of these areas, in my opinion, need one and the same home base if they are to be sensibly activated. Therefore, my major concern with the delivery system is with the primary or first point-of-contact care, known as **primary care** (see **Figure 4.1**), where perhaps as much as 80-90 percent of all health services can be rendered.[3] The reader must remember throughout this discussion that current-day operations described as primary care are often markedly different from those proposed in the classic source document of Parker[4] in this book, or in the literature.[5] It is of interest that self-help, with assistance from a properly organized primary care center, could even become the first level of care.[6]

My proposals are not Utopian prescriptions; they are normative ones. We may never agree on perfection, nor could we reach such a state even if we could agree on it. But we can design systems which move us towards generally desired states of affairs, where more people are more nearly self-determining, more fit to carry out their roles, i.e., are more healthy.

I. CARE AND CURE

This area of health care delivery focuses on the requirements for the more traditional health-related services. The prescriptive attributes of

FIGURE 4.1
LEVELS OF MEDICAL CARE

(Characteristics)	Primary	Secondary	Tertiary
1. Geographic Service Area (population base)	Neighborhood, local (pop: 2-10,000)	Sub-regional (pop: 100,000+)	Regional (pop: 1,000,000+)
2. Service Delivery Site	Doctor's office, general clinic, neighborhood health center	Specialist's office, general or community hospital	Usually hospital, as university medical school or special hospital
3. Personnel and Orientation	Family or general practitioners (first contact for care), patient-care oriented	Specialists (usually seen by referral), patient-care oriented	Super specialists (contact by referral), teaching and research oriented, limited patient care
4. Level of Skill and Technology Used	High level of skill in *general* patient care, screening level of technology used in diagnosis and treatment	High level of skill in *specific* patient care, specific level of technology used in diagnosis and treatment	High level of skill in very specific patient care, *very specific* levels of technology used in research, diagnosis, and treatment
5. Type of Care Given	Ambulatory, preventive, emergency, care for common diseases, referral to other levels of care for less common diseases.	Care for less frequent and less common disorders, more specific diagnostic and treatment needs	Care for rare and complex conditions
6. Continuity of Care	Continuous care, annual check-ups, preventive care, following through all levels and types of services	Less continuous care, patient returns to primary level after treatment for less common illness	Discontinuous care, patient recovers from illness and returns to secondary or primary care level
7. Quantity of Care	Major amounts of patient care given	Less than majority of patient care given	Small amount of patient care given
8. Cost of Care Per Illness	Lowest	Higher	Highest

[1]Sources adapted from A. Parker, M.D. "The Dimensions of Primary Care, Blueprints for Change," in *Primary Care Where Medicine Fails*. Edited by S. Andreopoulos, New York: John Wiley and Sons, 1974, and Bay Area Comprehensive Health Planning Council, Areawide Health Facilities and Services Plan, 1973. "Neighborhood/Local Services" and "Preventive and Maintenance Care," and readapted from P. Kelzer, Comprehensive Health Planning Association of Santa Clara County, November 1973.

[2]In rural areas, includes hospital care such as deliveries, appendectomies, simple fractures, pneumonia.

medical care that commonly are considered are shown in **Figure 4.2**. We shall go a bit further.

The individual's initial point of contact for well-being assistance must include, or be intimately associated with, all the major sources of somatic, psychic and social support, and control All facilities in which human services are offered cannot provide all potentially-relevant services. However, it will be argued that at the most commonly used first point of contact with health providers, the social, psychic, and somatic services should be together and be brought as close to those served as feasible (**Figure 4.3**). We will call such a service unit a **Primary Well-being Center** (PWC). Where the suggested variety of services cannot be physically housed in one site, all the services still must be related to one another in a clear and barrier-free way, as though they were part of one

FIGURE 4.2
CHARACTERISTICS OF GOOD MEDICAL CARE SERVICES

Available

Accessible financially, organizationally, and time/distance-wise

Acceptable with empathy for consumer outlooks and participation

Appropriate to family and community orientation

Adaptable to differing needs and over time

Comprehensive coverage

Continuity, and coordination of coverage and services for illness and wellness

Choice among services and providers

Equitable, in that care is provided in accordance with "evident" need, irrespective of means or cost

Efficient, safe, and effective technical application of services, i.e., affects health favorably, using suitable means of lesser cost when available

Quality, in terms of all the preceding factors

Accountability of the serving organization, in terms of assuring all the preceding factors

Adapted from A.W. Parker, *Personal Communication*

functional entity. This means horizontal connections in terms of primary somatic, psychic, and social care, and vertical connections in terms of relating the primary, or first point of contact care, with more demanding, more expensive, and less-frequently used therapeutic modalities of secondary and tertiary care centers. In some nations, including the U.S., many large groups of servers, as well as state-level, people-serving agencies appear to be moving in the direction of relating somatic, psychic, and social services at all service levels.[7] The generally overlooked but pressing societal demands made on medical care beyond caring and curing, such as social sorting and certifying, are also major uses of medical services which must be taken into account in organizing the PWC.[8] The capacities to deal with community-level issues is another inescapable aspect of the services a PWC must offer.[9]

FIGURE 4.3
CONFIGURATION OF THE HEALTH CARE DELIVERY SYSTEM AND THE MEDICAL CARE DELIVERY SYSTEM, WITH EMPHASIS ON THE PRIMARY WELL-BEING CENTER AND ITS RELATIONSHIPS TO INCREASINGLY-SPECIALIZED SECONDARY AND TERTIARY SERVICE CENTERS

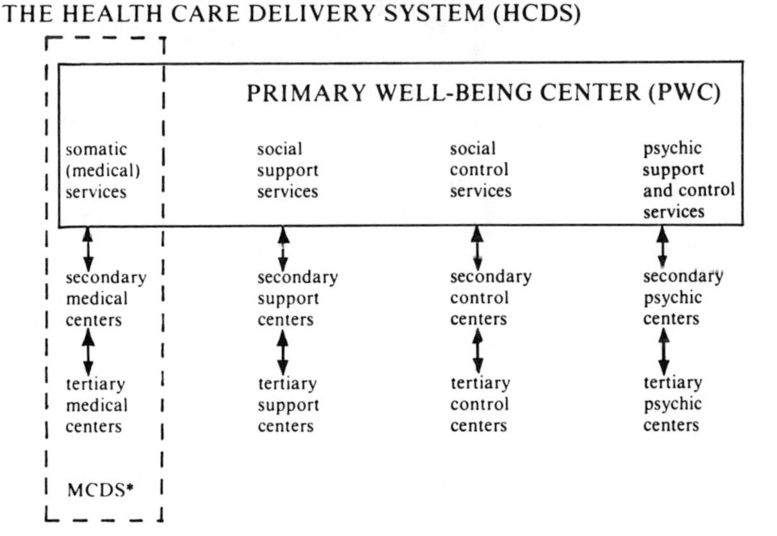

*The Medical Care Delivery System (MCDS)

Social control concerns Because some medical, and much of social and psychic caring, is associated with controlling, it seems desirable that the PWC should also include the partially-controlling and partially-caring parole-type social workers, whom I refer to as **social control agents**. Such secondary and tertiary level services are usually work, rehabilitation, or prison-type operations, although some of their tertiary centers are also hospitals in one way or another.

The psychic carers also use specialized secondary and tertiary centers. Whether acknowledged or not, these have **control** and **therapy** as their two main functions: social control may vary from high security isolation to simple supervision for part of a day, and therapy may vary from laboring to intensive supervised sessions of interpersonal interaction. These become very complex legal issues as well as social ones.[10] The patient neglect and confusion that has occurred because these loci of therapy have operated independently and have responded to the vagaries of shifting approaches do not always make for pleasant reading.[11]

The social control aspects of the medical care services are generally overlooked because they have more to do with sorting and categorizing to determine whether persons will be permitted to engage in certain activities. Admissions to some schools, to many jobs, and to professions are subject to medical scrutiny and approval (that is, control).

The control aspects of the social welfare services are often ignored, but they may represent the main stimulus for providing such services.[12]

Barriers to utilization must be removed One of the most vexing issues of putting client together with server is the complex set of interactions (see **Figure 4.4**) that take place to make suitable utilization of services a reality.[13] Financing, of course, has a critical bearing on determining who can enter the system.[14] The mode of financing also has a bearing on who utilizes services and who is willing to provide services to whom.[15] Obviously, the first requirement of an equitable care system is to remove the financial barriers. But, as will be seen later, how this is done will have remarkable consequences in many quarters that cannot be overlooked.

By examining **Figure 4.4**, we find a welter of interactions possible at each of the four loci, and between the four loci, that will affect utilization. Many of these, such as geographical access or cultural mismatches are quite as important as financing.[16] Even the process of utilization itself cannot be overlooked, for it sensitizes both server and served and is very likely to determine future relationships with other like participants. For example, will the provider be accepting of the Medicaid client's appearance and/or behavior? Will the provider be reimbursed suitably? Will the Medicaid client be accepted for care? And, subsequent to the care received, will the client ever again seek care except in desperation?

One highly-visible door for those who hurt or have a problem General systems theory tells us that any manifestation of ill-health may have its origins in social, psychic, or somatic system levels. We also know

FIGURE 4.4
FORCES AT WORK IN
THE UTILIZATION PROCESS

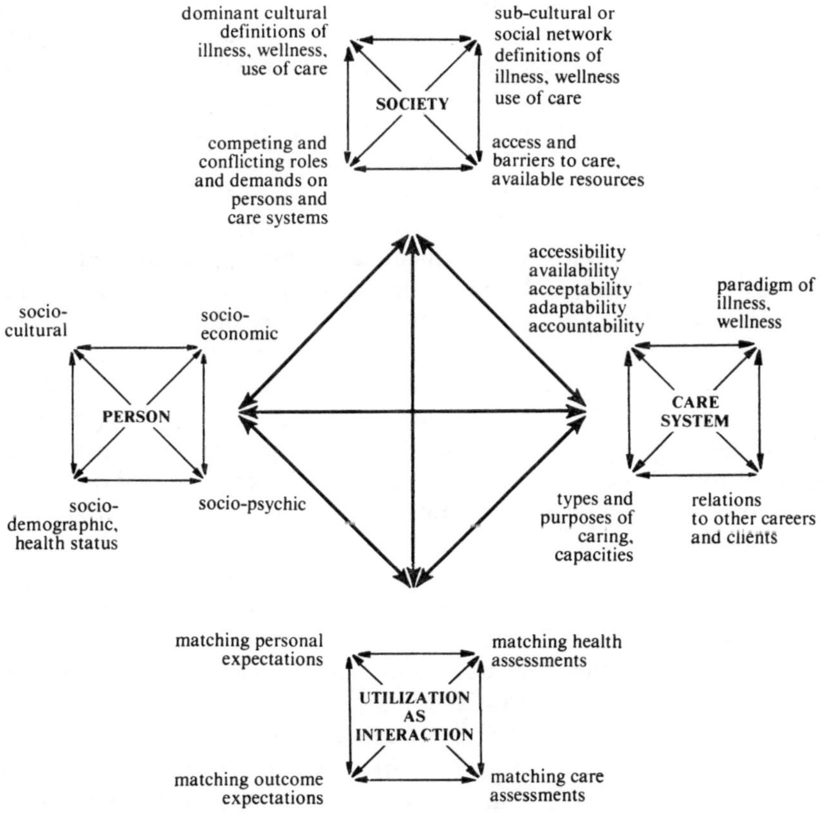

Adapted from H. L. Blum "Utilization in the Health Care Delivery System" in *The Social Welfare Forum, 1975,* New York: Columbia University Press, 1976, 98.

that no individual should be expected to unravel the mystery as to which of the servers to select. One most urgently needs the somatic helper if there is an ulcer which is hemorrhaging, but one also needs the psychic or social carer if the same problem is to be attacked at its point of origin. The same victim may need services from these and many other helpers, such as nutritionists or legal advocates, to overcome various obstacles to the restoration to reasonable health.

Given the necessary interrelatedness of the work, it is inexcusable to have each service isolated and unheedful of others, each with different admission hurdles, available only at different locations and at limited times.[17] By the same token, any health service door that is open must be so organized as to be "the door" to enter any of the PWC galaxy of services.

A single convener for each person or family It is of dubious wisdom to set the person with problems loose to wander among servers, none of whom need have the specified assignment of seeing that the resulting care is rationalized, that priorities are set, and that there is full comprehension and participation in care. There should be a single convener, no matter what the basic discipline, suitable for any patient with a significant complaint. It might be adduced that a person with a problem should be attached to a convener whose skills best match the apparent need. However, since a client has access to any required servers through the convener, and since the nature of the origin of most illnesses (even of fractures) is not all that clear, the discipline of the convener seems less important than his or her capacity to develop a helpful relationship with the troubled person. Unskilled conveners who need guidance from others on nearly all of a client's issues may not be too useful. Yet those of us having experience with so-called indigenous workers, who have minimal formal social, psychic, or somatic skills, observe that often they seem to be the only ones able to relate to difficult clients and bring them to participate in their own well-being. Perhaps empathy is just as important a server ingredient as a well-being discipline or skill. Biller makes the point that the uniqueness of the individual client forms quite a contrast with the norm-centered views of many of the health professionals. As a consequence, the latter have great trouble dealing with individuals. He therefore suggests that the convener should not have the narrowed outlook of any of the professionalized servers.[18]

The use of a multipurpose worker as a convener is a related issue which has been discussed many times, as has the use of a multipurpose or community-oriented primary care unit.[19] It is not our intention to review the utility of a multipurpose worker, except to point out that the laying on of hands to one client by five to 20 professionals from one to ten agencies, from any or all of the four service systems shown on **Figure 4.3**, with each worker acting in a semi- or totally-independent manner, is not conducive to assisting anyone with serious problems. Where, because of distance to a secondary or tertiary service, the PWC convener can no longer directly follow the client who needs such services, a convener at the secondary or tertiary level must take over the immediate convening duties in that setting and also relate back to the basic PWC convener for client return, client-family problems, follow-up explanations about informed consent,[20] and other matters. In centers where various of the PWC staff members form into a different (relevant) team for each client, it is understood that each client will have a convener assigned at the moment of entry to the PWC. As the patient's needs are unraveled and relationships clarified, a new convener (or the original one, if appropriate) becomes the team leader for that client, convening other services as indicated. The client also has the opportunity to shift to a more satisfying convener if and as the nature of concerns, desires, and requirements so indicate.[21]

The issue of client acceptance of servers other than physicians, in the health care setting, has been raised and answered repeatedly in straight-forward terms. Clients will accept those who treat them well; they will accept designated non-medical carers. They will also show individual preferences and biases. Since the envisioned PWC offers each client a choice and change of conveners, and true participation in his or her own care, this issue of client acceptance seems to be less than critical.[22]

All servers have a system view and are willing to share a client's care when indicated At such time as client well-being becomes the measure of successful caring, conveners and those who do a special task for a given person must share the care well and freely. For example, until there is comprehension of the possibilities as to why persons fail to keep appointments or neglect their health in one way or another, there is likely to be minimal care or it is likely to be misplaced. The pediatricians who do not want to care for poor children because of broken appointments and general neglect not only have to be concerned with the origins of "destructive" behavior but they must have access to the PWC team member who has the family's trust and has, or can activate, the skills needed to intervene at the social and psychic levels in order to get useful client participation.

Outreach is a necessity Many individuals are ignorant, many afraid, and many more feel unwelcome in places set up to care for problems. Not only do people delay in getting attention for serious problems, but many who do come in become so scared by the implications of the diagnosis, or so distrustful or alienated by the treatment they receive, that they do not return appropriately and do not carry out their treatments as prescribed. For these and many other reasons, it is often necessary to use indigenous outreach workers to seek out families suspected of not pursuing a healthful existence, of having members at high risk, or of having known problems. The outreach workers provide encouragement and assist families to carry out behaviors that are essential to their well-being.

II. MICRO-ECOLOGY: SELF-HELP, SELF-CARE, SHARE-CARE, AND HELP-OTHERS, AS SELF-ACTUALIZATION

This area is devoted to the extension of health concerns, away from what is done by the server for the served to primarily what clients do for themselves and even for others.

The individual is the unifying key through whom needed care, i.e. promotive, preventive, and therapeutic interventions, are channeled It has been suggested that *there are some health matters for which the individual has the basic responsibility to develop and maintain appropriate behavior, and for which the primary focal point of the health education interaction is at the level of the individual.*[23] It is this area that I would call **micro-ecology**.

A. In Health Maintenance and Heightened Reserve

We have already seen that in developed societies the individual's behavior is a key factor and, even if constrained by environmental forces, a potent means by which one's own health is to be maintained or improved (promoted). For example, if one is to minimize risks from cardiovascular disease caused by diet and inactivity, from perturbations caused by alcohol, drugs and tobacco, or from trauma generally, one will have to learn to pursue a different life and to enjoy behaviors and activities of which many were, and again could be, satisfying. This is **self-help.**

The same attitudes that promote living in moderation should be a reasonable base on which to build demand for protection against dental decay or anemia, to seek immunization against contagious diseases, or to develop awareness of roles played by social and psychic stress. In some cases, the protection is achieved by personal hygienic and dietary matters; in others, by checking with professionals on indication, or at appropriate times as worked out between the person and the health advisors. Satisfying and involving contacts at the PWC are seen as the brightest hope for promoting healthful behavior.[24]

It seems reasonable to think of being taught, of developing, and of being tested for personal competency in health as part of one's schooling. In a health center, without any element of compulsion, it would seem even easier to make better health-enabling behavior attractive to a significant portion of the populace. By a mixture of well-timed therapy for critical events, and preventive interventions at known stressful points in maturation, it also should be possible to assist individuals to strengthen themselves to face future rounds of perturbations.[25] The critical times in life that call for social or environmental advice and support are obvious for the infant, particularly the toddler, for whom the stage is set by producers of lead paint, by housing policies that generate or perpetuate slums, by manufacturers of flammable night clothes, by designers of dangerous toys, by parents who use pills and pesticides carelessly, and so on. A mixture of systems-conscious promotive and early diagnostic outlooks has become known as **Prospective Medicine.**[26]

B. In Early Diagnosis

Utilization of health services is dependent on learned client behavior, as well as on the availability of specific components of professional service. Individuals learn to seek advice, inspection, or assistance in the presence of suspected problems, or to come in for checks at certain times when it is well-known that certain hazards are likely to be encountered. Scrutiny for anemias of pregnancy, for cancer of the breast and cervix, or for hypertension are examples of necessary professionally-designed assistance in areas where, as yet, no other certain means of prevention or caring exist. This is **self-care**.

C. In Therapy

Taken ill, the client must be a co-venturer in care with the servers, and be as much in charge of his or her part of the intervention as is feasible. This is **share-care.** I do not discount the client's need for regression to a dependent stage and to heavy use of a convener in severe crisis, so that one can tolerate overwhelming pain, disability, and complex therapeutic regimens preparatory to regrouping his or her capacities. But I find it hard to agree that all care should be given by professionals outside the home, because "only the carer knows," or "because our tiny nuclear family in the U.S. is already overburdened to the breaking point."[27] The client often can and has to do much, if not most, of the therapy. One's recovery and continued well-being often involve maintenance and reserve strengthening also. He or she may have to learn such new techniques as meditation, or utilize bio-feedback to get in touch with his or her own systems.[28]

The client can, and often desires to, assist in the care of others with whom he or she is close, and be assisted by them in turn (**help-others**).[29] Not only does this help one comprehend the what and why of one's own illnesses, but focuses attention on causality and the need for future patterns of behavior that will aid well-being.

It is important to reiterate that the lay citizen's first line of defense is built on the ongoing education that enables one to use self-help intelligently (of course, if pushed to extremes self-help may become independent self-care, in which no professional advice is sought or tolerated). We are interested in the self-help and its extensions described in this section because it is self-actualizing. It builds a sense of confidence in one's capacity as well as in one's ability to negotiate with professionals. In all these situations, self-help, help-others, and share-care with professionals not only makes possible a lower cost of care and a wider coverage of services for all persons, but should make possible more appropriate services and a more intelligent utilization of them.[30]

In addition, this participation is seen as increasing a client's self-image, communications, and the capacity to work with others in a general environment of hopefulness and usefulness. The growth of self-help organizations among handicapped persons, and the scope of their functions, has been an eye-opener for professionals as to what self-help can produce and what it means to those with major health deficiencies.

Blaming the victim We must be clear that very little of human behavior is a purely voluntary matter. Behavior represents learned responses of an individual (or group) to an environment. It will not do to wash our hands of the person who takes up smoking, who fails to exercise, and who lives in front of television in spite of our admonitions. Nor can self-actualization techniques be expected to overcome massive macro-ecologic forces which produce undesirable behavioral micro-ecologic responses. "Blaming the victim" is a neat way of ignoring malfunctioning socio-economic systems and, with an easy conscience, letting the victims writhe who do not have the resources or who have not found the personal capacities to overcome the effects of such macro forces.[31]

III. MACRO-ECOLOGY: SURVIVAL WISDOM AND COLLECTIVE BEHAVIOR

A. The Source of Survival Wisdom

One element that keeps emerging in each area of requirement is the need for development of survival wisdom and collective survival behavior if the individual is to achieve more than erratic and temporary improvements in somatic, psychic, and social well-being. Speculations on where *homo sapiens* is going do not reflect sanguinely on how well *homo sapiens* is going to do, but clearly suggest the need for one to try to do better than one has.[32] The declining marginal utility of new medical technological breakthroughs, and their increasing potentials for iatrogenic damage, call for each individual's participation in his or her own care decisions, as well as in broad social decisions, about the development and use of many interventions.[33] Moreover, the extension, at great costs, of duration of life but not always of living, calls for even more public wisdom to set guidelines for the endless professional pressures for knowledge and fame, and the near endless societal pressures on professionals to "do everything possible."

The source of primary care must have the capacity and interest to attract persons for societal well-being concerns and survival wisdom To my mind, there is no easy alternative to using the primary well-being center and the health care system to involve and inform people about the critical need for their involvement in the survival affairs of their world. In this regard, it is important to note that consumer involvement is more likely to occur through use of, and participation in, good services than through the opportunity to participate in governance.[34]

A place to come for concerned talk The setting for primary care must offer attractive facilities for gatherings held under the auspices of various servers who have messages they want to deliver. However, some of these gatherings, preferably most, should be held as a result of the interests of well or sick members rather than at the initiative of professionals.

It does not seem too farfetched to imagine that a well-being center, located close to those it serves, known for the concern of its planners and governors (who are themselves recruited from the ranks of the served), and appreciated for its interest in individual and community well-being, could find support and talent when needed to aid its clients in acquisition of survival wisdom. Whether such efforts would result in political potency is another matter. How well various PWCs would complement or support one another, or even think of the same issues, is more problematical. They might conceivably end up before the political decision makers as competitors for limited resources.

The individual is the key through whom needed environmental or supra-system, health-promoting changes (survival wisdom) can be initiated In addition to affecting personal life-style and health-promoting behavior, the person affects his or her environment through behavior sparked by attitudes towards other people (social behavior) and towards the maintaining ecosystems (ecologic behavior).

Social and **ecologic behaviors** are critical to the long-range well-being of the individual's supra-systems, and thus to one's own and one's offspring's survival. While individuals learn about themselves, they also have to learn about the role of supra-systems and ecology in keeping themselves healthy. From this, he or she may learn to use influence politically, socially, and economically to redirect the societal institutions of which he or she is a directing and directed element.[35] Many persons are (and many more could be) attracted to the social participation that would help reconcile values and sort out alternatives for making the biosphere a more desirable and healthier place to live. A systems view illuminates the importance of involving individuals in the issues that they inevitably help shape, whether by action or inaction or by knowledgable or misinformed concern. What more logical use of the health care delivery system is there, particularly through its primary center, than to involve as many individuals as possible in looking at that larger scene? Through their experiences around their own hurts and their translations of the origins of ill-health, many could be involved in the future of their community and of their world. And it seems unlikely that there will be other comparably available or involving settings in which this critical new role for *homo sapiens* can be initiated on a broad scale.

B. Reconciliation of Micro and Macro Views of Intervention

Figure 4.5 points up the relatedness of how micro or individual efforts can be used to help create collective or macro efforts. In turn, macro efforts can be used to create individual efforts. The role of social support networks is seen as central to supporting efforts at both self-help and collective action.[36]

Routes **1-3-7** or **1-2-3-7** are those in which the individual responds to general concern, and can and does use efforts within one's own "wiggle" room to achieve a more healthful way of life. At the same time, the concerned individual can help generate collective action for those things that can only respond to collective action, e.g., **3-5-4-8.** One also can help in carrying out collective action, e.g., **7-9-8**. It is of interest that collective action undertaken in response to general concern also may be needed to help one help oneself, e.g., **4-6-3-7**.

FIGURE 4.5
RISK REDUCTION, MUTUAL REINFORCEMENT
OF MICRO AND MACRO APPROACHES
(UTILITY OF SOCIAL SUPPORT NETWORKS.
FOLLOWING PILISUK)

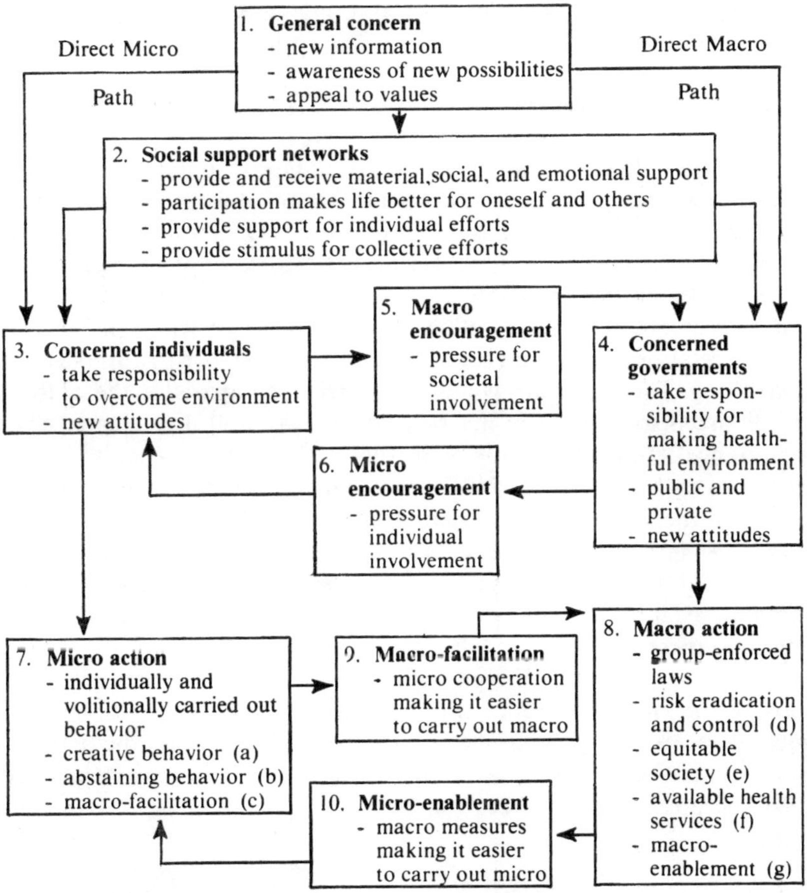

(a) =exercise, stress reduction, etc.
(b) =cease smoking, cut calories, etc.
(c) =cooperate with others to get better environments **7-9-8**
(d) =make safer, less toxic, less violent society, etc.
(e) =remove unemployment, poverty, etc.
(f) = rational organization of health services
(g) =help individuals carry out their own health improving tasks **8-10-7**

Adapted from "Social Perspective on Risk Reduction," H. L. Blum, *Family and Community Health*, 3:1, May 1981, by permission of Aspen Systems Corporation.

Thus we see that at the level of encouragement macro can support micro (**4-6-3**) and vice versa (**3-5-4**). Similarly, at the level of enablement or facilitation to take the necessary action, macro can enable micro (**8-10-7**) and vice versa (**7-9-8**).

The great argument about the relative virtues of individual self-help as opposed to societal or collective action seems to evaporate once we appreciate that we need great quantities of both if either is to take place. And both must take place if we are to overcome the risks which only society can stop and those in which the individual must not indulge. Because the level at which one intervenes is so critical, this issue shows up as a major planning consideration in **Chapter 8**.

C. Social Support Networks

The proper place in which to elaborate upon social support networks is not easy to determine. On one hand, it would seem to be little more than an extension of self-help (micro). On the other hand, it is clearly some form of collective action (macro), even if unintended. So, much as shown in **Figure 4.5**, it seems to deserve a place in both micro and macro. The importance of social support networks, or at least their high correlation, with better health and better resistance to adverse forces, is far-flung. The better survival of the married, compared to the widowed, the divorced, or the never-married persons, is well documented. Their importance in mental health or in illness prevention generally[37] seems particularly potent. The PWC, through each client's convener, can ascertain the closeness and usefulness of the client's existing support networks. The convener can help introduce the isolated client to many networks: those of like illness if one has a serious chronic one, those with common health interests, or those with common or potential social, political, recreational, or intellectual interests.

Clearly, among the particularly useful types of networks worth starting for and with clients, are those which work on PWC service or governance issues, general health issues of concern in the PWC, or general socio-economic issues which are of concern to many clients of the PWC because of their effects on health.

D. Resources and Control

This is the macro area of governance in which significant consumer involvement will have to take place if there is to be intelligent consideration of utilization and allocation of resources at the PWC.

Primary care delivery, and the total health care delivery systems of which they are a part, must be under consumer control The PWCs which horizontally tie together the major social, psychic, and somatic servers, and which vertically tie together primary with secondary and tertiary level services, call for heavy consumer input, if not control. Consumers must participate in all committee structures, from general planning to quality and utilization committees. Various reasons for consumer control and participation have been offered, such as decreased alienation, engagement of the sick person in a process which will lead to self-healing, creating neighborhood power, development of a constituency, countering the inevitably self-serving health professionals, and creation of more service alternatives.[38] Widely differing roles and degrees of consumer involvement, from utilization of services to full control, have been presented and debated.[39] My major concerns with consumer control are elaborated upon in **Chapter 5.**

IV. HEALTH EDUCATION IN NEW ROLES

The work being carried out at PWCs has many implications for changes in the outlooks of consumers and providers alike. The health education functions, epitomized by, but hopefully not limited to, persons having health educator training, are basic to the dissemination of the systems concept of illness and well-being to all subscribers of the care system. It is possible to describe the health education tasks required for each phase of the work done in the PWC.

A. In Care and Cure

In the realm of therapy, we have seen that the process of receiving care is complicated by many factors, too many of which are not understood by either the server or the served. A health educator is needed to structure the interchange sessions in which server and served have a chance to explore hang-ups occasioned by everything from personality to cultural and professional-client discrepancies.[40] In fact, even the modest variety of servers in a PWC will need to be interfaced in skillfully-arranged sessions with, and in behalf of, one or another client or type of client, because of the limited understanding each of the servers currently has of one another's conceptual outlooks, and of their typically-shared, limited understanding of human ecology and well-being.

At the same time, interfacings have to be arranged among consumers so that they, the consumers, can get a sense of why they have such divergent needs and demands, and why it will never be possible to do everything for everybody. This allows for the possibility of creating consumer groups whose members are at risk from similar circumstances or hazards (e.g., pregnancy, working unmarried mothers with young children), or those who are already coping with full-blown social, psychic, or somatic problems (e.g., diabetics, hypertensives, returnees from mental hospitals). An extension of this work goes into the self-help and help-others categories, already referred to previously.

Although presumably the work of conveners, the focus on clients' living needs may turn out to be a major role for health educators. The unbelievable disregard of providers for the disabilities and handicaps resulting from not-so-rare impairments is a major area of failure among physicians. A famous scientist's amazing tale of being allowed to go blind by the country's leading specialists, without one sentence being uttered on how to overcome some of his disability, is "must" reading for physicians.[41] Equally important are the physician practices of shutting off conversation by standing up stiffly while the patient is trying to get to some conclusion, or by handing out a prescription in lieu of relevant conversation or as a show of having everything under control.[42] Even more to the point are the physician pre-emptions of the patient's right and need to know about diagnosis and prognosis.[43]

The above examples are but a few among many problems that involve the relatively-unexplored relationships between servers and served that explain the parting of the ways between them. Each of us, as a patient, has one or more typical horror stories that we can tell about the totally unconcerned care we have received that makes a mockery of the "scientific" aspects of professional care. The reconciliation of the needs of servers and served will call for case-by-case review and interchange between the two. It will take a skilled health educator to turn these encounters into learning events that help both the server and the served.

B. In Micro-ecology

In the realm of promoting wellness beyond the issues of care for any current problems, the health educator will have a special role in arranging for the diversity of information-giving required by all ages and all kinds of persons. At the same time, the health educator must take on the more significant tasks of arranging for participation in the areas of nutrition, exercise, relaxation, developing better health habits, meditation, bio-feedback, caring for others, and so on. It is in these areas of doing things for one's self and for others that larger strides in creating wellness have to be taken. It is going to take energetic health educators to create awareness and to make consumer involvement possible with the support from providers.

C. In Macro-ecology

Again, it will take health educators with a well-developed sense of the systems hierarchy of *homo sapiens* to arrange for client exposures to the larger physical, socio-economic, and cultural environments that determine our locations and dislocations, our threats, our promises, and our opportunities. Health educators will have the responsibility for arranging the opportunities for clients and providers to enter into the issues of conservation, nuclear power, air, water and soil pollution, unemployment, housing, transport, and so on. It is individuals who create community awareness of the major forces that promote or threaten health, and of what can be done about the forces. PWCs have to provide the leadership for comprehension of the ecology of health, for there is no other relevant center offering an opportunity for involvement with health concerns.

D. In Governance and Planning

The PWCs need an internal source of stimulation and education to assist subscribers and providers in learning about their own planning and governance processes, as well as of the larger Health Care Delivery Systems of which PWCs are the central core. Health educators have the necessary background for bringing about these opportunities for discussions, for formal and informal education about group work, for organization, planning, and evaluation, and so on. Health educators are needed to arrange for exposures, even confrontations, between diverse consumers, between consumers and providers, and between diverse providers. It is only in these ways that differing value and belief systems can be placed on the table, and that the legitimacy of the differences made clear.

V. THE UTILITY OF PROMOTING WELLNESS STRATEGIES APART FROM SERVICES AT A PRIMARY WELL-BEING CENTER (PWC)

This issue is addressed by Mico and Ross, from a theoretical viewpoint based on Maslow's Theory of Self-actualization.[44] It does not conceptualize health as a harmonious interaction among the *homo sapiens* hierarchy of systems, and therefore does not necessarily see a well-being center as the place where their harmoniousness is promoted or restored. It is likely that proponents of a solely self-actualization approach would not want to be involved in a setting where the caring of illness also occurs. By contrast, the proponents of a general systems viewpoint would want both aspects to be interdigitated in what they regard as the inseparable work of minimizing ill-health, doing the most with what health one has, and promoting future health.

In fact, there are many examples of the wellness strategies now being pursued both in and apart from PWCs. It is my belief, however, that a center where both the hurts and the desires for better health can be answered has many advantages over the separating of the services for sickness from those for health or prevention.[45]

Each type of concern almost has to be built onto the others if there is to be any coherence to a person's health efforts. Those who seek illness care can be attracted to wellness care if both concerns are simultaneously promoted by the same source of care. Those seeking wellness guidance will also be better able to use illness care if the same center and servers are available, interested, and trusted.

Before leaving the issue of the nature of "good" system requirements, it is worth re-emphasizing how one set of descriptors of what is "good" health can lead to very different requirements in the eyes of different beholders. Alford describes how a system intended to do the "desired" things emerges differently from the belief systems of three sets of interests: professional practitioners, bureaucrats, and community advocates.[46] Freymann comes up with a totally different care configuration, even though he shares a good many desires and views in common with me.[47] Essentially, he takes the posture of professional practitioners and strongly believes in leaving the power in their hands, with modest inputs from non-professionals.

REFERENCES

1. P. F. Drucker, "Hysteria Over the Work Ethic," *Psychology Today*, 1973, Nov. 87-92. D. Mechanic, *Politics, Medicine, and Social Change*, New York, John Wiley and Sons, 1974, 261-270.

2. S. Toulmin, *Human Understanding*, Oxford, Clarendon Press, 1972, Vol. 1. N. Maccoby, et al., "Reducing the Risk of Cardiovascular Disease," *Journal*

of Community Health, Winter 1977, 3:2. K. G. Bauer, *Improving the Chances for Health: Lifestyle Change and Health Evaluation,* National Center for Health Education, San Francisco, 1980.

3. S. S. Bergen, Jr., "Primary Health Care: Suggested Organizational Structure," in *Primary Care: Where Medicine Fails,* by S. Andreopoulos (Ed.), New York, John Wiley and Sons, 1974, Ch. 4, 101-137. J. T. Hart, "Relation of Primary Care to Undergraduate Education," *The Lancet,* 1973, October 6, 778-780. K. L. White, "The Ecology of Medical Care," *New England Journal of Medicine,* 1961, 265, 885-892. K. L. White, "Life and Death and Medicine," *Scientific American,* 1973, 229:3, 23-33.

4. A. W. Parker, "The Dimensions of Primary Care: Blueprints for Change," in *Primary Care: Where Medicine Fails,* S. Andreopoulos (Ed.), New York, John Wiley and Sons, 1974, 15-76.

5. R. J. Gross, "Primary Health Care: A Review of the Literature through 1972," *Medical Care,* 1974, 12:8, 638-647. WHO, "Primary Health Care," *World Health Forum,* 1981, 2:3, 315-367. Institute of Medicine, *Community Oriented Primary Care,* Washington, D.C., National Academy Press, 1982.

6. J. Fry, "The Place of General Practice," *International Journal of Health Services,* 1972, 2:2, 165-169. A. H. Katz, "Self-Help Groups: Some Clarifications," *Soc. Sci. Med.,* June 1979, 13, 441-494. A. Gartner and F. Reissman, *Self-Help in the Human Services,* San Francisco, Jossey-Bass, 1977.

7. F. Baker, "From Community Mental Health to Human Service Ideology," *American Journal of Public Health,* 1974, 64:5, 576-581. F. C. Carlucci, "The Future Outlook for Delivery of Human Services," *Health Services Report,* 1973, 88:10, 891-893. *Directory of State Human Services Agencies,* Human Services Institute, Washington, D.C., 1974, July. R. Gumbiner, "FHP Pioneers Delivery of HOM Psychiatric Care," *FHP News,* Fall 1974, Family Health Plan, Long Beach, California. R. Gumbiner and R. Frye, "Management and Marketing in Health Care," *The Western Journal of Medicine,* 1973, 118:6, 65-72. J. T. McLeod, "Consumer Participation, Regulation of the Professions, Decentralization of Health Services," a report submitted to the Minister of Public Health, Saskatchewan, J. T. McLeod Research Associates Ltd., Regina, August, 1973. J. Hastings, *The Community Health Center in Canada,* Ottawa, Information Canada, 1972. N. A. Cummings and G. R. Vanden Bos, "The Twenty Years Kaiser-Permanente Experience with Psychotherapy and Medical Utilization: Implications for National Health Policy and National Health Insurance," *Health Policy Quarterly,* Summer 1981, 1:2, 160-175.

8. A. L. Childs, "The Functions of Medical Care," *Public Health Reports,* 1975, 90:1, 10-14. J. T. Shuval, *Social Functions of Medical Practice,* San Francisco, Jossey-Bass, 1970.

9. K. A. MacDonald, A. G. Hedberg, and I. M. Campbell, Ill, "A Behavioral Revolution in Community Mental Health," *Community Mental Health Journal,* 1974, 10:2, 228-235. C. Skrovan, E. T. Anderson, and J. Gottschalk, "Community Nurse Practitioner," *American Journal of Public Health,* 1974, 9, 847-853. The Southwest Health Centre in Indianapolis. The Aboriginal Health Centre, Central Australian Aboriginal Congress, Inc., Alice Springs, Australia, 1979.

10. R. C. Allen, "The Insanity Defense: An Uncertain Future," *Mental Health,* 1974, 58:4, 4-7. H. Blatte, "Evaluating Psychotherapies," *The Hastings Center Report,* 1973, 9, 4-6. D. Mechanic, ibid, No. 1, Chapter 13 and 14, 203-248.

11. F. N. Arnhoff, "Social Consequences of Policy Toward Mental Illness," *Science,* 1975, 188:4195, 1277-1281.

12. V. Navarro, "Social Policy Issues: An Explanation of the Composition, Nature and Functions of the Present Health Sector of the United States," paper based on presentation at the Annual Conference of the New York Academy of Medicine, April 25-26, 1974, Johns Hopkins University, Baltimore. F. F. Piven and R. A. Cloward, *Regulating the Poor: The Functions of Public Welfare,* New York, Pantheon Books, 1971.

13. H. L. Blum, "Utilization in the Health Care Delivery System," in *The Social Welfare Forum,* 1975, New York, Columbia University Press, 1976, 96-114. J. B. McKinlay and D. B. Dutton, "Social-Psychological Factors Affecting Health Service Utilization," in *Consumer Incentives for Health Care,* S. J. Mushkin (Ed.), New York, *Prodist,* 1974, 251-303. D. B. Dutton. "Explaining the Low Use of Health Services by the Poor: Costs, Attitudes, or Delivery Systems," *American Sociological Review,* June 1978, 43, 348-368.

14. R. Anderson and J. Newman, "Societal and Individual Determinants of Medical Care Utilization in the United States," *Milbank Memorial Quarterly,* 1973, 51:1, 95-124. E. Berkanovic and L. G. Reeder, "Can Money Buy the Appropriate Use of Services? Some Notes on the Meaning of Utilization Data," *Journal of Health and Social Behavior,* 1974, 15:2, 78-92. D. Coburn and C. R. Pope, "Socioeconomic Status and Preventive Health Behavior," *Journal of Health and Social Behavior,* 1974, 15:2, 67-78. K. Davis, "Financing Medical Care: Implications for Access to Primary Care," in *Primary Care: Where Medicine Fails,* S. Andreopoulos (Ed.), New York, John Wiley and Sons, 1974, Chapter 4. E. W. Hassinger and D. Hobbs, "The Relation of Community Context to Utilization of Health Services in a Rural Area," *Medical Care,* 1973, 11:6, 509-522. L. Montiero, "Expense is No Object: Income and Physician Visits Reconsidered," *Journal of Health and Social Behavior,* 1973, 14:2, 99-115. T. T. H. Wan and S. J. Soifer, "Determinants of Physician Utilization: A Causal Analysis," *Journal of Health and Social Behavior,* 1974, 15:2, 100-108.

15. H. L. Blum, ibid, No. 13. M. I. Roemer, et al., "Health Insurance Effects," *Bureau of Health Economics Research Series,* No. 16, Ann Arbor, Michigan, School of Public Health, University of Michigan, 1972.

16. L. Aday and D. Andersen, *Access to Medical Care,* Ann Arbor, Michigan, Health Administration Press, 1975. H. L. Blum, ibid, No. 13. J. B. McKinlay, "Some Approaches and Problems in the Study of the Use of Services: An Overview," *Journal of Health and Social Behavior,* 1972, 115-52.

17. E. A. Leopold and L. Schein, "Missing Links in the Human Services Nonsystem," *Medical Care,* 1975, 13-7, 595-606.

18. R. P. Biller, "Disaggregating Health Promotion and Health Care: Policy Initiatives that Depend Less on Homogeneity Assumptions and More on Human Uniqueness," prepared for Conference on National Health Policy, February 12-13, 1976, San Francisco, Working Paper No. 49, Graduate School of Public Policy, University of California, Berkeley.

19. H. L. Blum, "The Multipurpose Worker: A Family Specialist," *American Journal of Public Health,* 1965, 55:3, 367-376. H. L. Blum, et al., "The Multipurpose Worker and the Neighborhood Multiservice Center: Mutual Experiences and Implications of the Rodeo Community Center," *American Journal of Public Health,* 1968, 58:3, 458-468. E. F. Torrey, D. Smith, and H. B. Wise, "The Family Health Worker Revisited: A Five-Year Follow-Up," *American Journal of Public Health,* 1973, 63:1, 71-74. H. B. Wise, et al., "The Family Health Worker," *American Journal of Public Health,* 1968, 58:10, 1828-1838.

20. California Supreme Court, "Court Sets Consent Guidelines," *American Medical News,* 1972, 15:50, 1-3.

21. D. M. Dressler and K. B. Nash, "Project Team Organization and its Application to Crisis Intervention," *Community Mental Health Journal,* 1974, 10:2, 156-162.

22. J. C. Bjorn and H. D. Cross, *Problem Oriented Practice,* Chicago, Modern Hospital Press, 1970. D. L. Cowen and J. Sbarbaro. "Family Centered Health Care — A Viable Reality?" *Medical Care,* 1972, 10:2, 164-172. Martin Luther King, Jr. Health Center, "4th Annual Report, Jan.-Dec. 1970," Montefiore Hospital and Medical Center, New York, 1971. E. C. Nelson, A. R. Jacobs, K. G. Johnson, *Journal of the American Medical Association,* 1974, 228:1, 63-67.

23. P. R. Mico and H. S. Ross, *Health Education and Behavioral Science,* Oakland, California, Third Party Associates, Inc., 1975, 7, 176-179.

24. C. W. Douglass, "A Social-Psychological View of Health Behavior for Health Services Research," *Health Services Research,* 1971, Spring, 6-14.

25. G. Caplan, *Principles of Preventive Psychiatry,* New York, Basic Books, 1964.

26. "Prospective Medicine: Improving the Patient's Survival Odds," *American Medical News,* 1974, Sept. 2, 17-19. L. D. Robbins, "Health Hazard Appraisal: Comprehensive Personal Health Programming in Practice," Indianapolis Methodist Hospital Graduate Medical Center, Aug. 1967. J. LaDou, J. N. Sherwood, and L. Hughes, "Health Hazard Appraisal Counselling: Continuing Evaluation," *The Western Journal of Medicine,* March 1979, 130:3, 278-85. L. Breslow and A. R. Somers, "The Lifetime Health-Monitoring Program," *The New England Journal of Medicine,* 296:11, 1978, 601-608.

27. T. Parsons and R. Fox, "Illness, Therapy and the Modern Urban American Family," in *Patients, Physicians and Illness,* E. G. Jaco (Ed.), Glencoe Free Press, 1958, 234-245.

28. K. R. Pelletier, "Neurological Substrates of Consciousness: Implications for Psychosomatic Medicine," *Journal of Altered States of Consciousness,* 1975, 2:1, 75-85.

29. M. J. Lerner, et al., "Hospital Care-by-Patient: An Evaluative Look," *Medical Care,* 1972, 10:5, 430-436. A. H. Katz, ibid, No. 6. A. Gartner and F. Reissman, ibid, No. 6.

30. A. H. Katz, "Self-Help in Rehabilitation: Some Theoretical Aspects," *Rehabilitation Literature,* 1967, 28:1, 10-30. A. H. Katz, "Self-Help

Organizations and Volunteer Participation in Social Welfare," *Social Work*, 1970, 15:1, 51-59. A. H. Katz, "Self-Help Groups and the Professional Community," *The Social Welfare Forum*, 1975, New York, Columbia University Press, 1976, 142-153. Ibid, No. 50. C. E. Lewis, "Improving Access to Primary Care Through Reforms in Health Education, Orientation and Practice," in *Primary Care: Where Medicine Fails*, S. Andreopoulos (Ed.), New York, John Wiley and Sons, 1974, Chapter 2. Ibid, No. 53. "Informing Patients About Drugs: Alternative Designs for Prescription Drug Leaflets," Rand Publications, Santa Monica, California, No. R-2800-FDA as reported in *The Nation's Health*, October 1981, 5. G. Smilkstein, "The Educational Pelvic Examination," *The Journal of Family Practice*, 1981, 13:6, 932-933. C. Viedma, "Women's Dispensary," *World Health*, Feb.-Mar. 1981, 28-31.

31. W. Ryan, *Blaming the Victim*, New York, Pantheon, 1971. N. Freudenberg, "Shaping the Future of Health Education: From Behavior Change to Social Change," *Health Education Monographs*, Winter 1976, 6:4.

32. R. L. Heilbroner, *An Inquiry into the Human Prospect*, New York, W. W. Norton, 1974. J. Salk and J. Salk, *World Population and Human Values*, New York, Harper and Row, 1981.

33. J. Powles, "On the Limitations of Modern Medicine," *Science, Medicine and Man*, 1973, 1, 1-30.

34. J. L. Falkson, "An Evaluation of Alternative Models of Citizen Participation in Urban Bureaucracy," Program in Health Planning, School of Public Health, University of Michigan, Ann Arbor, Michigan, 1971. A. G. Motulsky, "Brave New World?" *Science*, 1974, 185-452. 653-663.

35. A. Ferguson, Jr., *National Health Proposals, the Neighborhood Health Center, and the Poor*, Neighborhood Health Center Seminar Program Monograph Series, Number 2, October 1971, University Extension, University of California, Berkeley. D. B. Dutton and J. L. Hochheimer, "Institutional Biosafety Committee and Public Participation: Assessing an Experiment," *Nature*, May 1982, 297:6, 11-15. H. R. Holman and D. B. Dutton, "A Case for Public Participation in Science Policy Formation," *Southern California Law Review*, Sept. 1978, 51:6, 1505-1534.

36. J. Fry, "The Place of General Practice," *International Journal of Health Services*, 1972, 2:2, 165-169.

37. C. B. Galiher, J. Needleman, and A. J. Rolfe, "Consumer Participation," *HSMHA Health Reports*, 1971, 86:2, 99-106. L. F. Berkman and S. L. Syme, "Social Network, Host Resistance, and Mortality," *American Journal of Epidemiology*, Feb. 1977, 109:2, 186-204. M. Pilisuk, S. Chandler, and C. D'Onofrio, "Reweaving the Social Fabric: A Model for Minimizing Against Stress Induced Illness," Table 1, Forms of Social Support Facilitation, Mimeograph, 1980, University of California, Davis, California. W. S. Breakey, "Community Support Systems and Urban Mental Health," *Urban Health*, November 1980, 31-34.

38. J. W. Guthrie, "Public Control of Public Schools: Can We Get it Back?" *Public Affairs Report*, Institute of Governmental Studies, 1974, 15:3, 1-5. N. Milio, "Dimensions of Consumer Participation and National Health Legislation," *American Journal of Public Health*, 1974, 64:4, 357-363. M. B. Mogulof, *Citizen Participation*, Washington, D.C., The Urban Institute, 1970, Jan. 1021-1.

39. S. R. Arnstein, "A Ladder of Citizen Participation," *Journal of the American Institute of Planners,* 1969, 35, 216-224. H. L. Blum, *Planning for Health,* New York, Human Sciences Press, 1974, 399-475. C. B. Galiher, J. Needleman, and A. J. Rolfe, "Consumer Participation," *HSMHA Health Reports,* 1971, 86:2, 99-106.

40. M. S. M. Watts, "Medicine and Society: Do We Need a Philosophical Reconciliation?" *The Western Journal of Medicine,* 135:5, Nov. 1981, 404-405. P. B. Heaton, "Negotiation as an Integral Part of the Physicians Clinical Reasoning," *The Journal of Family Practice,* 1981, 13:6, 845-848.

41. D. Stetten, Jr., "Coping with Blindness," *The New England Journal of Medicine,* August 20, 1981, 305:8, 458-460.

42. S. A. Wortman, et al., "Do Prescriptions Adversely Affect Doctor-Patient Interactions?" *American Journal of Public Health,* Dec. 1981, 71:12, 1358-9.

43. S. Godow, "Truth: Treatment of Choice, Scarce Resource, or Patient's Right?" *The Journal of Family Practice,* 1981, 13:6, 852-860.

44. P. R. Mico and H. S. Ross, *Health Education and Behavioral Science,* Oakland, California, Third Party Associates, Inc., 1975, 7, 176-179.

45. H. A. Schrier, "Medicine Versus Health: A Comparison of Two Systems," *The Pharos,* July 1975, 125-129. W. Winkelstein, Jr., "Is There an Alternative to the Holistic Approach to Health Care," paper presented at the Conference on National Health Policy Issues, San Francisco, Feb. 12, 1976, School of Public Health, University of California, Berkeley.

46. R. R. Alford, "The Political Economy of Health Care: Dynamics Without Change," *Politics and Society,* 1972, 2:2, 127-164.

47. J. Freymann, *The American Health Care System,* Baltimore, Williams and Wilkins, 1974.

Chapter 5

ONE EXAMPLE OF A DELIVERY SYSTEM THAT MEETS OUR REQUIREMENTS FOR EFFECTIVE HEALTH CARE

In this chapter we continue with the imagery of **Figure 1.1** (page **4**), and fill in the "institutions" shown in **Box E**. This chapter is devoted to describing the nature of 1) the overall health care system, 2) its four major sub-systems, 3) the primary well-being centers, and 4) the interrelationships of the segments to the whole, as portrayed in **Figure 4.3** (page **89**).

More detail will be directed to the medical or somatic services than to the psychic or social services during this discussion in order to provide a more tangible picture of one of the four major service areas that I am suggesting be combined in order to create an effective overall health care delivery system (HCDS). Moreover, the medical services are presently quite apart from the others, and there will probably be interconnection of the various medical elements long before widespread attempts are made to combine the medical with the psychic and social sciences, as we propose.

I. THE PRIMARY WELL-BEING CENTER (PWC)

The PWC is the client's home base. (I use the term **client** in preference to **patient** because it signifies an active, participating role rather than a dependent one, and does not imply that the user of the services is restricted to participating in the system only at the times when he or she feels sick.) The PWC serves clients in their initial or primary contact with care, and refers them as needed to secondary, tertiary, and other specialized settings (**Figure 4.3**, page **89**). Though the PWC has to carry on with technical medical decisions made for individual patients attending these secondary and tertiary level elements in the service hierarchy (**Figures 4.1** and **4.3**), it is the dominant or head unit in the sense of general patient supervision and policy setting for the entire system. The medical care servers in the PWC "share" their patients with at least three other service systems shown in **Figure 4.3**. At the lower levels (secondary and tertiary), the relationships of the four serving systems need not be particularly "tight" for other than improvements in exchanges of care, advice, and records.

I do urge that the primary care or head unit of all four delivery systems be solidly merged into one PWC, for five reasons: 1) essentially all of the inseparable well-person concerns can be determined at this center; 2) the bulk of all emergency, restorative, or supportive services of all four systems can be carried out here; 3) persons with a significant problem in one area generally require some services from one or more of the others at the same time; 4) when a person or family requires services at the secondary or tertiary levels in one or more systems, these can be kept sensibly organized through the PWC which acts as the client's home base;[1] and 5) the health or well-being of the community served is a central concern of the PWC.[2]

The distinguishing features of primary, secondary, and tertiary level somatic services were presented in **Figure 4.1**.

The patient or family relates to, and is guided by, one convener at the PWC For clients with anything more than the simplist episodic needs, I see it as indispensable that one PWC worker, whether at the outreach or professional level, be designated as the client's convener. The convener becomes the key support, source of advice, and supervision through whose intervention the bulk of all services from any of the four systems is arranged for the client. A full discussion of conveners was given in **Chapter 4**.

PWC staff, skills, and size Let us examine the scope of skills that is appropriate in the PWC so that it can render medical services, social support (i.e., social work and social welfare), social control (usually in the form of probation social work), and psychic support and control (usually in the form of mental health services, along with scattered efforts by other agencies, such as those concerned with alcoholism and drug abuse). PWCs can be of many sizes, but an upper limit of 10,000 subscribers seems reasonable. **Figure 5.1** provides one speculation about

FIGURE 5.1
PRIMARY WELL-BEING CENTER SKILLS AS EXEMPLIFIED BY PERSONNEL NOW AVAILABLE*

Skill	Personnel for 10,000 people	Personnel for 2,000 people	Primary center needs in U.S.	Total now available and active in U.S.
Basic Medical Care				
Family Physician[1)2)]	3	1	70,000	55,000 General Practitioners. 65,000 Internists. 24,000 Obstetricians 25,000 Pediatricians
Physician's Assistant[3)]	4	2	90,000	4,000.
Registered Nurse	3		70,000	1,250,000.
Licensed Vocational Nurse	3	1	70,000	650,000.
Dentist	4	1	90,000	135,000.
Dental Hygienist	2	½	45,000	40,000.
Dental Assistant	6	1	125,000	50,000.
Optometrist	1	½	22,000	24,000.
Optometric Assistant	1	¼	22,000	2,500.
Podiatrist	½	⅛	12,000	9,500.
Therapist	½	⅛	12,000	28,000 Physical Therapists. 14,000 Occupational Therapists. 10,000 Other.
Nutritionist	1	¼	22,000	30,000, of which 22,000 are Dieticians.
Pharmacist[4)]	1	¼	22,000	155,000.
Laboratory Technologist	1	¼	22,000	100,000.
Laboratory Aide	1	¼	22,000	30,000 basically unlimited; need three-12 months training.
X-ray Technician	1	¼	22,000	125,000.
Well-being Support				
Health Educator	½	⅛	12,000	25,200, of which 3,500 have MPHs and 20,000 are School Health Educators.
Health Education Aide	1	½	22,000	Unlimited supply, Associate of Arts level and six months training.
Psychiatrist	½	⅛	12,000	26,000.
Lawyer	½	⅛	12,000	
Legal Aide	1	½	22,000	Bachelors level and six months training, unlimited pool.
Public Health Nurse	1		22,000	50,000.
Social Worker	2		45,000	150,000 of which 20,000 are aslo shown under Mental Health and 10,000 are Medical Social Workers.
Mental Health Worker	2	4	45,000	34,000, of which 20,000 are Social Workers and 14,000 are Clinical Psychologists.
Mental Health Aide	2		45,000	150,000, of which 10,000 are probably appropriately trained.
Probation Worker	1		22,000	
Outreach	4		90,000	Unlimited, with brief training.
Environmentalist	1	½	22,000	Many kinds, pool very broad: at least 90,000.

1) Includes doctors of medicine and osteopathy.
2) One internist, pediatrician, or obstetrician equivalent to one family practitioner.
3) Nurse practitioners, or physicians' assistants of other kinds.
4) Not basically a dispenser of drugs: where that is included, need equal pharmacist aide time.

*Some data drawn from:
1) *Profile of Medical Practice,* AMA, Monroe, Wisconsin, 1980, 140-158.
2) *The Supply of Health Manpower,* USDHEW, Washington, D.C., 1970.

the skills needed in a PWC serving 2,000 persons and in one serving 10,000 persons.[3] Limiting service to 10,000 persons or less seems to be a real virtue, for it not only allows close proximity to those it serves but the smallness of staff helps keep bureaucratic structure and mechanistic relationships at a minimum.

Skills are listed in **Figure 5.1**, in terms of the types of personnel now available to convey the scope of tasks. But this does not mean to imply that these are necessarily the specific types of personnel that would be desired. Rather, the "packaging" of old skills, along with new ones, into new skill disciplines, seems logical and calls for a constant evolution of health worker types. (Changing nurse role expectations and frustrations, even in secondary and tertiary institutions, sacred to the physician rule, became evident as the major issue in the 1974 nurses' strike in the San Francisco Bay Area,[4] and continues to mount in intensity and unhappiness.) The work responsibilities of primary care workers also can be placed into the categories of independent, interdependent, and dependent in accordance with establishment of well-defined roles in a given PWC.[5]

Figure 5.1 also indicates the total numbers of such workers that would be needed if every person in the U.S. were affiliated with a PWC, and contrasts that number with the estimated numbers of servers in each category who are now working at related tasks. This does not mean that all persons in a given category are freely available now. But, with few exceptions, it does indicate that not only do we *not* have shortages of the manpower required but that we are probably utilizing significantly more manpower in scattered services and on unnecessary services than would be required to do a good job based on full primary care coverage.[6]

The feasibility of shifting less technical duties to less extensively trained or more generalized personnel is being intensively explored now. The evidence indicates tremendous potential for enlarging the scope of services by such means, as well as the hazards of introducing more fractionation.[7]

Finding, reorienting, and relocating presently underused medical servers into the underserved areas, in a group or team setting, is being explored in many areas. The success of such relocation seems highly associated with the absence of pre-existing, well-established, older forms of medical practice.[8] However, the successful conversion of most obstetricians and internists, even pediatricians, into more general primary or family practitioners is unlikely. Fortunately, it is not necessary.

More vigorous attempts to direct a higher proportion of new health careerists to primary care and underserved areas is discussed briefly in **Chapter 6**.

All related primary, medical-related services belong in the PWC
All of the medically-related services, such as dentistry, optometry,

pharmacy counselling (preferably, but not necessarily, filling prescriptions), podiatry, various therapies, and nutrition counselling are essential parts of primary medical care. It is not imperative that all these servers be physically located in the same facility, or be intrinsic partners or employees in a unitary organization. But they must be part of the PWC and be bound by a set of common financial, administrative, and service commitments to a given group of clients. In any one organized delivery system or PWC, some servers may work on a contract, some on fee-for-service, some on salary, some on special incentive programs, and so on.[9] But in every PWC it is important that each of its servers be easily available to its clients, identifies with all the other servers of that PWC, and knows how to reach and use them in behalf of their mutual clients.

The team, and "who will have the last say?" The burning issue that keeps tumbling out from the more status-conscious servers is, "who will have the last say?" in any such new scheme for care. Physicians are used to having this prerogative and most can't conceive of its being otherwise. Yet in their own medical environment, they constantly share decisions with more specialized physicians, nurses, social workers, psychologists, and other technologists.

In a PWC, the convener shares decision making with the client, and they both share it with other experts as these are called in.[10] There is no "permanent captain" of the team. The role of the convener is the closest there is to being captain for any one client, but each other expert server may take temporary captainship for a special event with the client. There is no fixed team, no super-leader, with the final word on all clients. In view of various experiences and surmises, this may be too glib an answer, but it indicates the direction to be taken.[11] One thing is certain: staff and patient relationships maintained solely by pecuniary arrangements will add precious little to good care.[12]

In order to keep the PWC operating, there will be a professional administrator to focus all operations, obtain equipment, keep staffed, obtain evaluations, hear and pursue complaints, and so forth. This does not give that person any special say about the nature of services to be offered to any one client. Likewise, this does not necessarily give him or her the highest salary, the biggest office, or the most status. The administrator has to help the servers and their clients get their job done effectively, if he or she is to have any status at all. The model of the non-medical-trained hospital administrator seems to be an appropriate one for the PWC. Undoubtedly, there will be many unexpected shifts in the roles of staff as a result of how the clients come to share in the structuring and the utilization of services.[13]

One of the key figures in the PWC will be the health educator, whose role in extending mutual awareness among consumers and providers will make the new functions proposed for the PWC possible (see **Chapters 4** and **6**). The micro-ecologic and macro-ecologic aspects (including governance) of consumer involvement, which are the keys to better health, better user utilization of care, and control of service costs, simply won't come about without assignment of an applied behavioralist to epitomize this set of concerns and to bring them off.[14]

Every person should have the opportunity to belong to one PWC located close at hand The services of a PWC should be made available to every person within the territorial limits of the U.S. This is not to say that each and every person must use these services. Other operations, including the present ways of providing services, would not be ruled out.

Multiple competitive PWCs in denser population centers In areas with sizeable populations there should be many competitive primary care groups, provided that each offers a full set of services, including ties to suitable secondary and tertiary units. Patients should have a choice among primary care units, whether the PWCs are parts of a single complete delivery system or relate to different complete delivery systems.

Multiple PWCs may co-exist in one physical structure In areas with dense populations, there is no reason to avoid placing multiple primary care units in a single structural setting, particularly when they are sister parts of one larger HCDS. Each would still have its own clients, and each client would have his or her own PWC and the freedom, within reason, to change to another. Even competitive primary units belonging to different delivery systems could be located in a single physical structure, even to sharing highly specialized equipment or skills.

It would be possible for such specialized servers as dentists, pharmacists, optometrists, therapists, and laboratory technologists to work in small isolated groups that act as technical resources to any one or many PWCs. This might simplify relationships among the servers at the primary care unit because there would be fewer of them housed in the PWC. However, it might also complicate relationships of clients to servers, as many of the servers not based in the PWC will become isolated or non-participant in the consumer and provider activities and attributes being developed at the PWC facility.

PWCs can be housed with secondary or tertiary units In large population centers, there is no reason why the primary unit or units cannot be located with, or be a relatively intrinsic part of, a secondary or even a tertiary unit. This will work under the proviso that the clients' basic care is always organized and guided by the primary unit, which is seen as the brain and soul of the well-being enterprise as well as being the site where the vast majority of all services are carried out.

Primary medical care should not be built up out of medical specialties I see it as totally unwise to deform the primary medical-care services (no matter how large the population served or how large the aggregation of servers in one location) into medical serving units built around teams of medical specialists. The non-primary care physicians should be in specialty departments or units, and should not be part of the primary or point-of-first-contact units. These specialty units are set up in appropriate numbers for the small percentage of medical conditions needing care at the secondary and tertiary settings.[15]

Variations in the service capacities of PWCs (and HCDSs) The amount, but probably not the scope, of all helping skills required will no doubt vary with client composition. The truly well-to-do and the majority of middle-class persons, who may be the first and strongest users of PWC-type services, may need a different mix of services than the poor. They will probably need less of the direct economic and social support services, but may be regular users, even if less ill, of most of the other services. How much they will become involved in the self-help, help-others, governance, survival-wisdom type of activities is problematical. They are heavily into the help-others and governance areas in the present health care settings. But these activities presently are not meant to be educational, nor are they carried out so as to be health improving.

The PWCs (and HCDSs) that get caught up in the excitement of making systems knowledge work for them may well need other skills than the basic ones already described. Sociologists, anthropologists, ecologists, and systems theorists will be needed and can be obtained; they probably are not needed permanently or full-time. Working relationships with colleges and universities can provide part-time expertise and lead to a sharing of accumulated knowledge in return for the opportunity of the educational center to do further studies and to train students.

II. THE MEDICAL CARE DELIVERY SUB-SYSTEM (MCDS) CONFIGURATION, WITHIN THE OVERALL WELL-BEING OR HEALTH CARE DELIVERY SYSTEM (HCDS)

Although we in no way encourage the isolation of the MCDS from the larger well-being directed HCDS, it is, for purposes of clarification, useful to look at the MCDS sub-system by itself, for a moment.

The elements of delivery of medical care must be tied together into a sub-system of the overall health care system, which can assure the resources, proper distribution of services, reasonable efficiency and effectiveness, basic quality, and easy entry to all elements of care. The medical sub-system must provide automatic connectivity, and transport where needed, for access to all other required services in the complete health care system, no matter where they are located. Such a medical care sub-system (**Figure 4.3**) must be able to create a suitable organization out of manpower, facilities, technologic instrumentalities, and financing.[16] The sub-system's clients and subscribers are partners in setting policy as to how the system is to behave, as well as being partners in acts of care, curing, and social sorting. A very hesitant gesture of support for the concept of comprehensive organizational structuring of medical care services has been made by the U.S. government, in P.L. 93-222, known as the Health Maintenance Organization (HMO) Act of 1973. Subsequently, more positive support has been legislated nationally.

Minimum MCDS size It seems unlikely that the functions described for an MCDS would be carried out very well in systems serving less than 50,000 persons. However, it may be that there is not much to be gained by systems serving over 100,000 persons, since an MCDS need not be the exclusive user or owner of secondary hospitals, therapy centers, diagnostic centers, nursing homes, tertiary care centers, and so on. These can be free-standing entities, serving many MCDSs on a contractual base. MCDSs, serving large groups, may create or acquire the specialized units, but few will ever be so large as to have all tertiary services, some of which require a population base of several million people in order to provide enough cases of rare conditions to enable a highly-specialized service unit to operate effectively and efficiently.

The MCDS sub-system is based on its primary care concerns and PWCs The primary care units, and the majority of the medical care functions carried out there, should be the key concern around which all other medical care in the MCDS is organized. Hospitals and medical care centers should not be the dominant interests, even though they may continue to swallow a major share of dollar resources spent by any one medical delivery system.

MCDSs may have many relationships with and between the servers in it A delivery system need not be one in which every server connected with it is an employee or partner. Servers may have a variety of such arrangements with the system as participation in governance, resource sharing, and client care, provided the system as a whole does the things we have outlined for it. The Independent Practitioner Association (IPA) type of HMO is an example of such a system which utilizes all types of servers. The collection of servers bound by contract guarantees the nature of coverage to be provided on an annual prepaid basis. Physicians and other servers continue to work as individual entrepreneurs or institutions under specified contractual obligations to one another and to specified consumers. Organizationally, an IPA is quite loose, but medically it is effective, with a tight level of money control and with a growing concern for knowing what is transpiring among its services and for improving quality.[17] Since it usually has minimal consumer participation in policy setting, it will be interesting to see when and how that can be introduced. One would guess that major consumer involvement should be easier to develop here than in the "closed panel" structured medical care delivery entities, such as Kaiser-Permanente. One such large HMO or MCDS has been controlled by consumers since its founding in 1947.[18]

Every person should be covered by an MCDS The aggregate of MCDSs in a region or a state should provide primary, secondary, and tertiary coverage for every person living in the area. Care should also be assured in every MCDS and PWC for travelers whose cost of care will be the responsibility of their home-base system, or of the federal government if they are citizens of other countries. Only in this way can we assure all persons in the U.S. of access to medical care at all times.

More than one MCDS may be operative in an area Once MCDSs are able to meet minimum size, coverage, connectivity, and efficiency requirements, there is no reason why several may not co-exist independently, offering consumers choices between systems. In fact, more than one in an area seems desirable.

Federal, rather than state, guidance is required A national set of minimal requirements for access, coverage, and quality of outcomes is required if we are to assure a basic level of care for every person in the land. The requirements should encourage opportunity for choice in all areas capable of supporting more than one MCDS. By means of national policy and laws, the hopelessly-conflicting state laws regarding licensure, insurance, and other barriers to reasonable care can be leveled. This still permits MCDSs to meet or exceed national standards in innumerable ways, in order to overcome or take advantage of indigenous population needs, resources, climate, and geographic attributes. In addition, there will have to be national policies on payment for professional education, distribution and placement of manpower, and so on.[19]

Federal gathering and redistribution of financing is required There are no ways in which poor localities or states can meet the cost of basic care requirements. Moreover, poverty will continue to shift from state to state, as will migrations of poor people. If the Reagan Administration's initiated cutback of federal taxation means that most federal money goes to armaments, then there can be no redistribution between states. If, in addition, states enact legislation restricting their capacity to raise money (e.g., Governor Reagan's ill-fated Initiative #1, in California, in 1973, which subsequently became the successful Jarvis-Gann Proposition 13 in 1978), there will be no way that states can help their poorer communities. Moreover, states and localities never have the money-raising capacities of the federal government.

For both ease of raising funds and redistributive reasons, the federal government is the best single center for gathering and assuring financing for all. It must do so at least on behalf of the poorest 25-35 percent of the population who usually cannot buy care, prepaid or otherwise. The inadvertent transfer of funds from poor to rich states, brought about because Medicaid requires state matching of federal funds received, has to be avoided;[20] as does the transfer from poor to rich individuals by consumer payments under Medicare,[21] which are financed by payroll deductions (on the first few thousand dollars of wages) and not at all from other sources of income.

All of the medical care funds on behalf of one person have to be in one MCDS The entirety of funds required and available for the medical services of any one person or family must be in a fund available to the MCDS, which contracts to cover the entirety of each client's needs for an annually-designated prepaid sum of money. It is only in this way that the MCDS, under consumer control and oriented to primary care, can allocate the resources where they are needed to effectively promote and maintain health. The current mis-allocated medical care dollars are directed excessively to secondary and tertiary care. Since currently there are few MCDSs and minimal producer or consumer awareness or concern for the basic care we envision at the primary level, little of it is produced. Moreover, for lack of primary care as part of a total MCDS, the secondary and tertiary levels inescapably expand endlessly, doing primary care expensively, as in emergency rooms, and caring for neglected and advanced conditions. Because each element of care is now delivered by an independent fee-for-service producer, the preventive and health promotion elements of care, for which insurance or governmental funds are minimally allocated, continue to be ignored.[22]

A single pool of funds available to an MCDS is also imperative if there are to be significant shifts of tasks to new skills. Only by overall MCDS decision making can it be made apparent, and worth the while of each producer, to consider other skills or modes of services. The substitution of optometric services for the physical optics part of the ophthalmologist's duties, the substitution of the optometric assistant's services for the optometrist's glass fitting, the use of physicians' assistants, and so on, commence to make sense once everyone is aware of the need to make a fixed sum of money cover all needs. Thus, less expensive and often equal or more satisfying modes of service become of interest.

The same pressures and possibilities created for the MCDS by one pool of money must be applied to the PWCs. In that way, psychic or social service substitutions for somatic or medical services commence to be worth scrutiny if it turns out that people can be kept healthier by non-medical interventions than by medical ones (and vice versa).

Licensure for MCDSs should begin to replace licensure for individual practitioners One of the major barriers to using new skills are the limitations placed by each state on the functions of each discipline as a part of its licensing requirements. These, of course, have always been promulgated by the various types of providers who mean to secure their turfs in that way. As a result, changes in the duties of a discipline, or the creation and utilization of a new one, poses a major legislative undertaking. Defined and licensed disciplines that are potentially affected fight changes; other disciplines not yet directly involved, feeling that precedents will be set, do likewise. The opportunities for PWCs, MCDSs, or HCDSs to experiment with new types of personnel are very modest and legally risky unless they can be given both the authority to create and use the new skills, and the responsibility, via licensing and outside evaluation, for guaranteeing the quality of the results produced by them.[23]

III. ACTIVITIES AND STRUCTURES OF THE NON-MEDICAL WELL-BEING SERVICES IN A COMPLETE HEALTH CARE DELIVERY SYSTEM

The preceding discussion of medical care, and of a medical care sub-system, can be used as a guide for what needs to be done equally about social welfare, social control, and mental health services. It is also important to remind ourselves that the major improvements in health are going to be obtained by major changes on the economic, educational, behavioral, and environmental fronts, which are closely related to the social and psychic services.

Each of the three major non-somatic, well-being, support systems, to be described, must be parts of a whole HCDS, in terms of the interrelationships with one another and with medical care. **Figures 4.3** and **5.1** illustrate how primary well-being centers might be structured and staffed with workers from the four major well-being support systems.

The three major non-medical health support sub-systems will be described only briefly, since their configurations are not seen as grossly different from the one for medical care. Because the secondary and tertiary services in the social and psychic areas are overwhelmingly governmentally-produced at present, their relationships to their counterparts in the PWC often will be different from those described for the somatic services.

Social support The PWC social resource workers, in addition to providing direct care services and arranging for in-home supports, would relate to secondary and tertiary social institutions, and organize appropriate levels and paths of care for individual and family clients. Welfare monies, housing services, and counselling are services that would be made available at the determination of the primary unit workers, who have the responsibility for assisting and guiding clients through crises or helping with lifelong incapacities. The client use of secondary and tertiary services, such as boarding homes, institutions for the aged, job training, and so on, would be arranged by primary unit workers.

It is not necessary to assume that only the social-work-designated person must minister to clients' social needs. Other members of the PWC could do it for most clients for whom they serve as conveners. However, the person specially skilled in social welfare might act as the immediately-available consultant for all PWC clients with complex social needs, and could offer direct services on a referral basis for clients served by other types of conveners. Similarly, the social worker often could be the major source of many other services for persons for whom they act as convener because social services were the clients' main need.

Social control The social-control oriented primary workers (i.e., probation workers), in addition to providing direct social services, would relate to secondary and tertiary control units, such as police, courts, jails, or penitentiaries, where the more enforcing and restraining tasks would continue to be carried out. But the pre- or post-incarceration guidance (i.e., probationary) tasks would remain with the PWC worker. It is not necessary to believe that only the probation worker can minister such required services. But the probation worker would be the resident expert for advising all other team members facing complex problems of delinquency. He or she could be the convener as well as the major dispenser of many well-being services for the client whose main needs are related to social control.

The traditional law enforcers are seen as the secondary level of social control in this schema. Their physical presence at a PWC might put the PWC "off-bounds" in the eyes of many disadvantaged persons. This comment does not mean that the PWC serves as a shield for law breakers, but since its concern is for maintenance or improvement of well-being it perhaps should not be identified with the law enforcer's image. (However, law enforcers have been successfully incorporated in the Britannia Center in Victoria, B.C., Canada.) Similar arguments have been made in regard to probation workers. However, the author's experience in working with such workers in a multipurpose center does not bear this out. Moreover, other social workers, even nurses, can be deputized to do the official probationary-type social work. Hopefully, such assignments would result in providing as much of a helping service as a controlling one.

Other extensions of social support The PWC staffing is designed to render somatic, psychic, and social care. How far can it profitably go in extending well-being support? Are employment, training, and counselling on civil and legal rights also services that can be offered here, or are they to be regarded as secondary, specialized resources to be kept apart? One can guess that not all PWCs would need such services, but those that serve a significant number of the disadvantaged may not be able to function effectively without them. Their presence in many Canadian service centers, and in the Southeast Health Center in Indianapolis, is considered to be central to meeting well-being needs for many clients. It would seem unwise to accrete other services, such as religious counselling and formal education, since these services already have major centers of their own which generally are highly visible, acceptable, and easily accessible. This is not to interdict cooperative PWC relationships with them.

Psychic support and control (Mental Health Services) The primary care mental health conveners would retain basic responsibility for their clients. In addition to providing direct services, they would relate to a mental-health set of secondary and tertiary resources, such as special treatment, residential, recovery, and half-way facilities in behalf of their clients. They would provide, or be the vehicle for providing, many of the related services for the persons whose main problems were emotional and for whom they were the conveners. Also, they would be the mental health resource for other PWC servers.

The often isolated services offered to drug abusers, alcohol abusers, retarded, and so on, should be as much a part of the functions of the PWC as any other support needed for victims of imbalances among the various systems levels in the *homo sapiens* hierarchy.

IV. PWC AND HCDS ACTIVITIES AND STRUCTURES REQUIRED TO IMPROVE CARE AND GENERATE MACRO AND MICRO HEALTH-ENHANCING MEASURES AND ATTITUDES

The interrelationships of servers and served in the proposed health care delivery setting calls for: 1) increased lay and professional comprehension of the nature of health; 2) wiser use of social, psychic, and somatic interventions in the light of where they seem most relevant, 3) demystification of the somatic and psychic services; 4) redirection of resources now necessarily expended on somatic manifestations to more on health education and self-involvement, thereby correcting behaviors that lead to massive ill-health; and 5) encouragement of political activity motivated to changing the behavior of various sectors of our society and major institutions towards support of a more healthful society.[24]

The large number of clients and servers who can work on committees, planning groups, and governing boards have a remarkable opportunity to come to grips with the interrelatedness of somatic, psychic, and social forces, and interacting systems. A major task of PWC planning committees will be to unravel the origins of common health problems coming to the PWC, and to work out the ways in which they can be prevented or solved. The need for putting this type of public health expertise into the local medical care units is being acted on in Great Britain.[25]

Even larger planning and governing tasks go on at the HCDS delivery system level, and at regional and state health planning bodies and health authorities. Obviously, the bulk of opportunities for participation are the ones closer to home, and each PWC should conduct a vigorous campaign to get clients and workers to serve in these functions.

Several Canadian proposals represent the beginnings of a new era of planning for care and for avoidance of health-damaging forces on a systems-oriented base.[26] Although other countries have done exciting health-promoting programs, the Canadians are among the first to look at what systems logic requires to be done if long-term well-being improvements are to be made in a developed country.

A. At the PWC Level

Governance at the PWC level Since the PWC is where well-being concepts are put to work, I believe it is imperative that those served provide most of the governance.[27] In addition, the PWC governing body receives advice from providers, guidance from the four systems of which it is the key joint venture, requests and complaints from consumers, and the hopes and recorded realities of how its subscribers are doing and how its services are being used. Such issues as the mode of selection of the governors, staggered and fixed-limit terms, issues of representation by social, race, sex, age (or preferably from organized, special consumer-interest groups, such as the aged, poor, parents, gay, Raza, Black, Native American, women, disabled, and so on), as well as other factors, have to be worked out in each PWC. Broad national guidelines must be provided to assure that these institutions work under participative democratic auspices that reinforce equitable practices (although such guidelines must not get into excessive detail). Unfortunately, there can be little delusion that the development of successful, heavy consumer involvement, as we envision it, is going to be a simple matter.[28]

Consumers must come onto governing boards from organized-interest groups in significant part (the way most providers do), for as individuals, consumers have a limited and evanescent stake or interest in health issues.[29] There are great needs for training consumers as they take on these new governance roles. Happily there are some effective pioneer efforts available for guidance.[30]

Planning for the PWC The never-ending function of planning for the PWC has three major objectives: that of achieving reasonable levels of health for its subscribers; that of making easily accessible to them a reasonable scope, quantity, and quality of acceptable health services; and that of maintaining a reasonable cost for its services.

What has been said about consumer involvement in governance applies equally to planning, for it is at the planning level that the goals and the means of reaching them should have the most clarifying examination.[31] The majority of those involved in planning must be consumers, but all vested interests must be on hand to make clear what they, the producers, know and worry about, and why.

There is a critical but generally-ignored need to hear from the non-consuming consumers in particular. For it is they who represent the failures of delivery or utilization that so plague us. It is from them that we learn whether services are unavailable, unaccessible, unpalatable, or meaningless. These non-consumers may constitute a sizeable minority, and may be footing their fair share or more of the costs of the system that they do not use.[32]

Likewise, the victims of extensive health failures, who have consumed heavily and widely, are heard from infrequently. Yet they have been the most prolongedly, diversely, and heavily impacted of all users; they could relate volumes about continuity, harrowing or satisfying episodes of care, and so on.

Somewhat related are the issues raised by consumer concerns, such as the Patient's Bill of Rights of the American Hospital Association and the significantly-expanded Denenberg Bill.[33] The right to decide on what is to happen to one's person, to an accounting on one's bill, or to reasonable courtesy, consideration, and privacy, hardly constitute a novel addition to the rights of a person who is purchasing a highly personal service. If these were not improvements over the existing state of affairs it would be ludicrous to proclaim the intention of letting the consumer have a particular subset of normal rights long vested in the individual by our laws.[34] But given the present state of affairs, these are important changes.

So let us move on to real consumer participation, so that such travesties in the name of restoring rights do not continue further into the eighties.

Understanding the forces that determine health, and their ecologic interrelationships, provides a remarkable educational opportunity for all who are engaged in planning. The services of a professional planner to assist in bringing out and reconciling a diversity of interests seems reasonable if not imperative, particularly in the early stages of exploring how to use the planning process. The services of a professional health educator seem equally indispensible if there is to be an expanding awareness or learning experience on the part of consumers and providers.

Quality control "Quality of health services" means how well they promote, maintain, or restore health. Quality control, in its most professionally-touted form of peer review (i.e., internal or self-regulation by the professional providers), obviously has gotten us to where we are. Essentially, peer review is devoted to technical proficiency rather than to what-care-does-for-health or how caring it is. Where the technical level of care is elegant, peer review works magnificently or, to be exact, has almost no meaningful work to do. Where it is most desperately needed, it doesn't, and hasn't, worked meaningfully. Without consumer participation in quality review, even professional incompetency is often swept under the rug of peerism. To the professional, the concept of quality usually is restricted to the technologic competency of professionals, and not to any of the other aspects of caring, or to what the services do for health itself, or for client independence and participation in self-help (micro) or in creating a more healthful environment (macro).

Utilization control Peer review to control unneeded utilization works reasonably well only in situations where there is full prepayment for a specified group of subscribers into a central financial pool out of which all providers are paid. This is true whether doctors are on salary, per-capitation, pre-allotted sharings, or fee-for-service basis. In the first three forms of payment there is no point in generating needless utilization particularly not if incentives are also built in so that there is distribution to the servers of any net savings generated by limiting the services they give; the major danger is that servers will do too little. In fee-for-service out of one total prepaid pool, it is to the interest of every server to make certain that no other server does needless work, thereby reducing the pot unfairly and "cheating" the other servers.[15]

More important than any of these concerns with control solely by vested interests is the need for control by consumers. Wasteful and sometimes dangerous abuses and over-uses of services by ignorant or incompetent consumers (or those from other cultures) are a major problem in most health care service systems. Experience indicates that controls over unwise consumer utilization of care cannot always be done effectively by the providers of services. The servers have never satisfactorily controlled client over-use, not even when applying their favorite remedies of financial penalties, such as co-payments (these also tend to deny services to the sick poor and to discourage preventive services). Only by being able to bring user profiles before the consumer-controlled governing body, so that consumers can see how individuals and groups under-use or over-use a service or fail to follow through, is there likely to be meaningful (health relevant) concordance established between users and servers. Those who are socially or physically ill and in need of assistance of other sorts may require supportive control available only from a user-run organization, where social incentives help the errant users to "fly right."

It is clear also that when serving systems are run by vested or producer interests, there has been little incentive until recently to seek out and bring in individuals and groups who dangerously under-use services. Most systems do not use outreach or even identify the under-users. Where the servers operate under an open-ended, fee-for-service scheme, as is typical with Blue Cross-Blue Shield, or commercial health insurance, or on the basis of fees paid directly by clients, there still exists an effective barrier to seeking out under-users in the form of the so-called "ethical constraints about soliciting business." In fact, it was not too long ago that even sending reminders to patients about "return dates" marked the practitioner as a hustler. The combination of hard times and newer marketing concepts are taking a hand in changing such views. In any case, the current poorly-coordinated maze of health care services provides no way to spot under-users except through surveys. Usually, only voluntary agencies and health departments carry on searches for under-users. But these searchers are typically desultory, under-financed and disliked by most private practitioners, and usually they are only for one or two health conditions.

Participation in care (self-help, share-care, and help-others) The serious involvement of persons or families in PWC activities that clarify how behaviors impact on well-being can lead to significant changes in how PWC members live. If the servers are heavily involved in leading the way, not only do they affect their own habits, they also set the stage for client participation in more self-care.

Clients can take more responsibility for their own medical, psychic, or social care routines once these are demystified and once professionals clarify what they hope to see happen. As this occurs, the client moves into a position of sharing responsibility for his or her own behavior and for overall decisions about the care one is to receive. By hearing and by being asked to respond to the servers' impressions the client can evaluate riskly procedures and life-changing routines with a good understanding on which to base decisions. It is only where consumers are treated as incompetent that they become controlled.

The professional's use of problem statements in family-linked problem-oriented records that include somatic, psychic, and social problems (which may be shared with clients), facilitates share-care as well as escalates professional and client understanding of supra-system influences on well-being.[36]

In the absence of the extended family, simple self-services can be taught to the client that do not call for visits by paid staffers. Where these visits must be arranged, "friendly visitors" can be trained to give them at no or little cost. In disadvantaged neighborhoods particularly, payment for these small services can help someone else be independent, and save the community money while providing timely, acceptable, and morale-raising services to incapacitated persons.

Let us help each client to take as much responsibility as he or she she is able. Let us increase, not decrease, one's doing capacity, one's image of one's capacities, and one's understanding of what one needs to be doing for his or her own welfare and for societal well-being.[37]

Because all interventions are attempts at setting up perturbations in one or another *homo sapiens* systems level, the patient as well as the server must understand their potentialities. Interventions can be unexpectedly potent, and they may do more than counter-act the problem-producing force or its consequences. They may over-act or under-act, miss the target entirely, or have independent side effects. The sharing of knowledge about the capacity of somatic, psychic, and social interventions to cause unexpected systems imbalances (iatrogenic diseases) could be educational for served and server alike. (See **Chapter 3**, on iatrogenicity.)

Formal consumer education Where levels of client general education are high, health is better. We do not know how general education influences well-being, or whether both of these attributes are affected by other independent variables. In any case, wherever the educational process goes on it is generally feasible to introduce health-promoting services and ecologic comprehension of health so that individuals are favorably influenced towards personal, health-promoting behavior. PWCs can take a hand in introducing and structuring the health education that can be made available to their members via the community schools as part of the general education offered there. Some carry on basic, as well as trade, education, e.g., the Aboriginal Health Center in Alice Springs, Australia.

Specific health education efforts will be needed in each PWC to carry out effective care-and-cure, micro-ecologic, macro-ecologic, governance, and planning activities. **Chapter 4** provided a discussion of the basic need for health educator expertise in order to conduct a systems approach to enhance well-being, a need held in common by provider and consumer.

Continuing professional education and training in the PWC In a dynamic setting like the PWC there will be a need for continuous updating of all skills. Fortunately, most of the PWC servers act as conveners for many clients. This task begins with a careful attempt to gauge the origins of each client's needs and to seek out relevant interventions. The ensuing sharing of clients with other skills, and the evaluation of successes and failures, with organized support, could be a continuing staff learning experience about the origins of good and bad health.

By combining the clinical training of student servers with the continuing education of the servers at the PWC, the various teaching centers can bring dynamic learning to servers, student servers, and clients. Students are particularly effective in raising embarrassing, forgotten, or over-looked issues, such as questioning services that don't seem to help clients. Faculties brought to the center to help put the social, psychic, and somatic disciplines together functionally at the level of caring for one client would receive tremendous stimulation from, as well as bring it to, the PWC servers who share the task of teaching students. Each has something different to offer the other. Professional education is treated in more depth in **Chapter 6**.

B. At the HCDS or MCDS Level

Governance The envisioned health-promoting delivery system would provide its clients with a remarkable array of services. There are many options for the specific governance of such systems at these levels. I would repeat essentially what was proposed in the way of governance for the PWC level; the critical considerations to which governance must be directed follow.

A given service unit must serve and be accountable to a defined population (subscriber) group Although implied by almost all of the "requirements" specified in this chapter, it remains to be emphasized that few of the requirements can be implemented unless there is a specified contract between a given service, such as PWC or HCDS, and a defined group of people who have contracted to be a part of it. Irrespective of how much choice people have, unless they assume the contractual role of subscriber and potential user of a given service entity, neither they nor the entity can find out what is going on with the subscribers or how suitably the services are designed; neither can the consumers or providers plan together around the nature and quality of such services for preventing, caring, or curing.

If there is no specified consumer-producer relationship, the idea of consumer choice and consumer control are essentially meaningless, since alternatives will have to be organized solely by the providers. Service units are likely therefore to be close replicates of one another. Providers, by themselves, can afford few risks on organizing and "selling" health promotional or preventive services; by being poorly organized for such purposes they further discourage a set of services already unappreciated by consumers. This would still be true even if preventive services were included in prepayment. Similarly, the problems of under-utilizers, over-utilizers, and the use of outreach workers would be undermined, since without contractual obligations the providers, as at present, would have no regular awareness of the members of any group or of the many care-delivering systems they use for various parts of their care.

An equally critical need for a defined constituency as the base for organized delivery units derives from concern with promotion of survival wisdom and behavior. Participation in the investigation of the sources of their illnesses, and production of the personal, social, and political behavior needed to alter perturbing influences in their lives, seem heavily dependent on the involvement of a specified group of persons receiving services from an organization they support, plan for, and govern with an eye to improving their own well-being.

Planning for the HCDS Like planning at the PWC, planning at the HCDS level is a never-ending, consumer-dominated effort that calls for a full-time planning staff. Among other things, its four sets of sub-systems each have to learn how its affairs inevitably affects that of the other sub-systems, and how the entire HCDS affects, and is affected by, all other aspects of society.

Non-partisan and consumer control of resource allocation between well-being sectors, service levels, categories of services, and manpower categories As long as vested interests, such as producers, manufacturers, insurance carriers, and government (Medicare and Medicaid) guide the decisions about the nature of resource allocations between sectors, we will have endless battles built around choice of interventions that will be settled more by the "war chests" and prestige of the interests involved than on the demonstrated utility or type of need. Inside the medical care sector, we have ample evidence of how service has shifted away from where people are and goes into the more expensive, and currently prestigious, secondary and tertiary centers. Not only is the training of primary care personnel a sometime thing which is again declining,[38] but traditional teaching-center research obscures patient concerns in the tertiary centers, and manpower is trained not for where the needs are but for the areas in which the trainers feel competent: witness the over-production of surgeons and other medical specialists.

Until there is consumer control there is almost no chance of creating HCDSs or PWCs that will do the job outlined here. What few good HCDSs and PWCs there are have come about as the result of institutions and legislation promoted by combinations of consumers, philanthropists, special situations, and maverick physicians who fought professional and other vested interests for years before they could legitimize their product.

The time for consumers to negotiate with their carers is not when they are ill and perturbed over their illness; nor is this the time when the sick person's family can try to make suitable agreements about quality, costs, or choice. Under the present purveyor-run services, the consumer can hardly bargain or stipulate anything, for once illness has occurred the patient or family is too vulnerable to dare question what the system has to offer.

Resources for serving well-being needs have to be in one pool As a corollary to what has just been postulated, it is essential that all resources for health services be in one place and be open to reallocation by one set of decision makers for a given group, such as the subscribers to an MCDS (HMO). On the surface, the trend to put all state-level, governmental, people-serving agencies together in one super agency suggests the possibility, if not the intent, of so doing.[39] The importance of this move becomes evident when we consider the following three considerations.

1. **Horizontal resource shifts at the primary level of care** At the start, the consolidation of the traditional serving agencies would bring together the various resources of manpower and dollars allocated for social, psychic, and somatic services at the primary, or point-of-first-contact, level. Pooling these resources, and working out how they take care of needs in the new conjoint setting will call rapidly for shifts in duties and in reassignment of personnel from one type of service to another. The tremendous changes that have appeared in medical practice as the result of the utilization of physician assistants is an example of shifts that can be expected at the primary care level.

2. **Vertical resource shifts** Tying together resources between the primary and the secondary and tertiary levels in each of the major well-being serving areas (prisons might be left out of the discussion at this time) will be necessary for the same reasons ascribed to

medical care. That is, the proper location of the services should be dictated not by where the most resources have been amassed but rather in accordance with what users and professionals work out as being the best arrangements for the effective use of the serving capacities and the insights we now possess.

3. **Resource shifts between sectors** The shifting of perceptions as to what are the major causes of poor health and well-being are bound to occur rapidly under systems scrutiny. For example, resources that are now used for medical care or penal surveillance in expensive tertiary institutions, might well be redirected to correcting such social perturbations as overcoming limited opportunities for disadvantaged groups. These shifts in the use of resources can be made only if all well-being funds are treated as a whole, in a central pool. Naturally, no single primary well-being center or health care delivery system can ever hope to amass this authority unless it is part of a nationally-approved approach to dispensing resources for well-being services at lower levels.

The concept of block grants for all human services, from the national to the state level is, in my opinion, a step in the right direction, although the problems are many.[40] Unfortunately, in the U.S., under the Reagan Administration, the block grants carry fewer and fewer resources. At the same time, the increased taxing for military purposes leaves no new taxing territory for states or city and county units. Moreover, those too poor to raise taxes get no helping hand even if they have the heaviest loads of ill-health.

All this is unfortunate, for block grants will become associated with disaster in the well-being area, for the wrong reasons. The block grants will be damned because we will associate them with **no resources,** rather than with their ability to allow resources to be moved about more intelligently to fit more locally-defined needs.

Throughout the country, in part encouraged by block granting, state and local governments, which operate the bulk of the social welfare, social control, and psychic support and control services, are bringing these pieces together administratively "at the top" into one human services entity. And a few are seriously contemplating their functional merger in the field into a type of PWC.[41] In addition, the somatic care services offered by state, city, and county public health departments and health care services are also being merged into the same overall human services agencies. Where tertiary-level institutions typically are a function of state government, as in mental health, local government is commencing to work in a more systematic way with the state to put related services into a vertically more coordinated financing and service posture.

However, still totally unintegrated (except for the large sums of money being paid to them by government in behalf of certain categories) are the private medical servers who provide the largest part of medical services. In fact, many government agencies that once created their own medical services now contract with private profit or non-profit producers to provide them. The need for medical care, and thus for the private medical sector to form or become part of rational systems for care, such as MCDSs, has been presented. The medical care systems, as well as the public-sector combined-services systems, offer no exception to the rule that all well-being services should be governed by those served. At the same time, the technologic wisdom and personal views of the providers should be considered an indispensable input. Like the governance of PWCs, many decisions will have to be made about reasonable representation, not only by types of consumers but by all types and levels of servers. The latter might best be dealt with by advisory boards of technologists, as most voluntary hospitals now have.

Variations in the "ownership" of PWCs and HCDSs The PWC could be a governmental, or a private non-profit, or profit-making organization. The possibility that a private for-profit operation would comfortably house person-centered, well-being, philosophic-political activities, and the psychosocial support and control services, is more unlikely than it is inconceivable. Given the level of entrepreneurship in the U.S., it is indeed likely that very complete and high technical-quality systems could be put together for profit purposes.[42] However, this would seem to rule out most consumer control, which I regard as key in promoting well-being. Consumer cooperatives are successfully into the provision of somatic care, and are one form of non-profit organization that can be expected to enter the HCDS field. Government-sponsored MCDSs (HMOs) are few and far between: the pioneer is the one created by the County of Contra Costa, in California.

V. INSTITUTIONS SEEM INEVITABLE: CREATING INSTITUTIONS THAT SERVE AS TOOLS OF THE USERS

New insights, new technological discoveries, and new problems will continue in an endless stream. They must be examined and acted on in the course of seeking better roads to improved well-being. Can this take place without institutionalization of the organized means to bring it off? We are all too painfully aware of the truth of Illich's position, that basic institutions such as education and medical care have fallen into the hands of those serving in it.[43] Irrespective of whether intended or comprehended, they minister more to their own needs than to those of the clients; above all, they cater to an affluency, growth, technology, consumption model which creates increasing dependency as well as social polarization. As another result, no one can enter the ranks of the servers except on their terms. Those who cannot use the providers' services, because of poverty or disagreement with how the system works, often must still contribute to it. And if they fail to use it they may be further stigmatized for the lack of participation. They may even have to create their own clinics, at further expense, to get (often non-reimbursable) the care they want. The evidence surrounds us, thanks to medical leadership, that we act as though medical care were the only way to attain better health. Yet, the evidence is clear that the present level of medical care is a terribly-expensive, too-little/too-late way of improving health status.

How do we counteract the dire prediction that institutionalization of such things as the HCDS and its PWCs is likely to prevent significant change, and that society will promulgate bad or useless things as the result of giving primary attention to the beliefs and desires vocalized by its institutionalized servers?[44] Perhaps we should first ask whether there is any way of improving our health status that could avoid the use of institutional forms. Currently, most North Americans very much want access to safe and good services for sickness, at costs which will not bankrupt them. They want a system whose costs can be controlled, with services routinely available around the clock. These services must be available and reasonably accessible to all, and be offered in a manner acceptable to many kinds of persons. The services they want are highly complex, and their wants cannot be met without massive organization (institutionalization).

We grant that all but a small percentage of the citizenry remain blinded by the institutionally-promulgated, illusory health promises of medical care; even to the point that their survival is prejudiced by their remaining unaware of other factors about their lives that could be harnessed by both individual and group non-medical actions to improve their health status. However, why can't we set up institutions that don't fall into the hands of those who are paid by them? If a place were made in the health care delivery institution for all Americans to act as adult *partners* in the care applied to them, and if they took a dominant role in that planning and governance, a more-realistic perception of what is involved in improving health status might develop; and institutional take-over by its workers might be avoided. Moreover, if there is no institutionalized system designed to reach and share care and governance with them, how will the populace ever come to an appropriate level of health insight and behavior?

Institutionalization seems inevitable for another reason. As much as we will promote self-help, share-care, and help-others, we will find it hard to approve the unlicensed practitioner (the level of whose skills has not been tested) to operate a Wasserman parlor, cancer therapy center, or whatever, because of one's individual rights or because we want more unfettered competition. I imagine that we will continue the institutions by which we now guarantee the competency of the provider (although by more rational ways than we now use) for the protection of the user who can never become sufficiently knowledgeable to make reasonable judgments about the adequacy or safety of those health services. The user may be a child, or an ill or handicapped person, or senescent adult who cannot make reasonable judgments about the need, desirability, or safety of a service. I hear all the arguments against institutionalizing the denial of the use of any quack or nostrum to the competent adult, but I can't believe that our society can look the other way, saying, "It's your choice, God bless you." So long as some choices are transparently dangerous to survival, and so long as our society knows that it will be asked to deal with the damage caused by incompetent care, such as supporting the victims of dangerous or inadequate services, and possibly their families, for the rest of their lives, there is social justification for institutionalizing the means of assuring that services offered to the public are as safe and as effective as we can sensibly make them.

In the interest of public safety, we cannot settle for a grand, anarchic, laissez-faire posture in the name of competition or of liberty of action for each person. This is no different in principle than allowing the wanton disposal of dangerous chemicals. We are all our brothers' keepers or murderers, as well as our own, and we have no choice but to help build the health framework within which we can learn how to promote our own well-being and how to understand the required limits to our liberties.

There is no out but to create the kind of institutions that will bring opportunity for people to participate in promoting their own and the general well-being, institutions that promote questioning and that facilitate changing.

It is also of interest to see what evidence can be mustered to suggest that *homo sapiens* or any other species has ever existed successfully without forms of institutionalizing. All four of Laszlo's attributes of natural systems presented in **Chapter 2** suggests that systems theorists see no evidence that surviving systems can be anything but sell-organized or institutionalized. My own limited search in this area suggests that the history of *homo sapiens* is most distinguished by the inevitability, variety, and comprehensiveness of human institutions.

I accept the inevitability of institutions. Therefore, I have described the requirements for, and have given an example of, an institutional framework for promoting well-being that should allow maximal opportunity for client control and education, the production and dissemination of new knowledge, and, above all, the opportunity to restructure health serving institutions as needed in order to apply new knowledge about well-being.

REFERENCES

1. F. C. Carlucci, "The Future Outlook for Delivery of Human Services," *Health Services Reports,* 1973, 88:10, 891-893. R. Morris, "Welfare Reform 1973: The Social Services Dimension," *Science,* 1973, 181, 515-522.

2. K. R. MacDonald, A. G. Hedberg, and L. M. Campbell III, "A Behavioral Revolution in Community Mental Health," *Community Mental Health Journal,* 1974, 10:2, 228-235. C. Skrovan, E. T. Anderson, and J. Gottschalk, "Community Nurse Practitioner," *American Journal of Public Health,* 1974, 64:9, 847-853. Institute of Medicine, *Community Oriented Primary Care,* Washington, D.C., National Academy Press, 1982.

3. J. C. Bjorn and H. D. Cross, *Problem Oriented Practice,* Chicago: Modern Hospital Press, 1970. A. W. Parker, *The Team Approach to Primary Health Care,* Neighborhood Health Center Seminar Program Monograph Series No. 3, January 1972, University of California Extension, Berkeley. A. W. Parker, "The Dimensions of Primary Care: Blue Prints for Change," in *Primary Care: Where Medicine Fails,* S. Andreopoulos (Ed.), New York, John Wiley and Sons, 1974, Chapter 1. R. L. Penn, Jr., The Application of a Model for Health Care Services in a Rural Setting," *American Journal of Public Health,* 1973, 63:1, 33-36, H. B. Wise, et al., *Making Health Teams Work,* Cambridge, Ballinger Publishing Co., 1974.

4. *Hospital Tribune,* "Nurse-Practitioners are Demanding and Taking Greater Responsibility," 1974, April 22, 8:9, 1-2.

5. E. Brunetto, "The Primary Care Nurse: The Generalist in a Structured Health Care Team," *American Journal of Public Health,* 1972, 62:6, 785-794. D. Wagner, "Nursing in an HMO," *American Journal of Nursing,* 1974, 74:2, 236-239.

6. J. P. Bunker, "Surgical Manpower: A Comparison of Operations and Surgeons in the United States and England and Wales," *New England Journal of Medicine,* 1970, 282:3, 135-144. E. F. X. Hughes, et al., "Surgical Workloads in a Community Practice," *Surgery,* 1972, 71:3, 315-327. G. S. Perrott, "The Federal Employees Health Benefits Program: Enrollment and Utilization of Health Services, 1961-68," HSMHA, USDHEW, HEW, Washington, D.C., 1971.

7. J. C. Bjorn and H. D. Cross, ibid, No. 3. A. S. Golden, et al., "Non-Physician Family Health Teams for HMO," *American Journal of Public Health,* 1973, 63:8, 732-736. A. Komaroff, B. Reiffen, and H. Sherman, "Protocol for Paramedics: A Quality Assurance Tool," *Quality Assurance of Medical Care Monograph,* RMP, HSMHA, DHEW, Feb. 1973, 161-178. R.

K. Tompkins, "The Role of Medical Audit in the Definition of the Quality of Patient Care Rendered by Physicians' Assistants," *Quality Assurance of Medical Care Monograph,* RMP, HSMHA, USDHEW, Feb. 1973, 139-160.

8. M. I. Roemer, J. A. Merd, and W. Shonick, "The Ecology of Group Medical Practice in the United States," *Medical Care,* 1974, 12:8, 627-637. Institute of Medicine, ibid, No. 2.

9. B. Abel-Smith, "Value for Money in Health Services," *Social Security Bulletin,* 1974, July, 17-28. D. Mechanic, *Politics, Medicine and Social Science,* New York, John Wiley and Sons, 1974, Chapter 18, 279-291.

10. R. E. Bouchard, et al., "The Patient and His P.O.M.R." *Quality Assurance of Medical Care Monograph,* RMP, HSMHA, USDHEW, Feb. 1973, 233-240.

11. J. I. Bufford and D. Kindig, "The Next Two Years," Institute for Health Team Development, Montefiore Hospital and Medical Center, New York, 1974. C. E. Lewis, "Improving Access to Primary Care Through Reforms in Health Education and Practice," in *Primary Care: Where Medicine Fails,* S. Andreopoulos (Ed.), New York, John Wiley and Sons, 1974, Chapter 2. Montefiore Hospital and Medical Center, "Institute for Health Team Development," 1972, Nov. 13, mimeograph.

12. J. M. Metsch, A. Schwartz, and W. Donn, "An Assessment of Provider Behavior in Shared Professional Facilities," *Public Health Reports,* 1974, 89:4, 307-314.

13. J. S. Beloff and M. Korper, "The Health Team Model and Medical Care Utilization," *Journal of the American Medical Association,* 1972, 213:3, 359-366.

14. P. R. Mico and H. S. Ross, *Health Education and Behavioral Science,* Oakland, California, Third Party Associates, Inc., 1975, 7, 176-179.

15. S. S. Bergen, Jr., "Primary Health Care: Suggested Organizational Structure," in *Primary Care: Where Medicine Fails,* S. Andreopoulos (Ed.), New York, John Wiley and Sons, 1974, Chapter 3.

16. K. L. White, "Primary Medical Care for Families—Organization and Evaluation," *The New England Journal of Medicine,* 1967, 277:16, 847-852.

17. D. C. Harrington, "The Relationship of Quality Surveillance to Various Health Care Delivery Systems," *Quality Assurance of Medical Care Monograph,* RMP, HSMHA, DHEW, Feb. 1973, 67-82.

18. H. S. Luft, *Health Maintenance Organizations: Dimensions of Performance,* New York, John Wiley and Sons, 1971, 13. H. S. Luft, *Health Maintenance Organizations,* New York, John Wiley and Sons, 1981.

19. Ibid, No. 1. D. Mechanic, "Some Notes on the Future of General Medicine Practice in the United States," *Inquiry,* 1973, 6:2, 17-26. M. I. Roemer, J. A. Merd, and W. Shonick, ibid, No. 8.

20. B. C. Stewart and L. A. Bair, *Health Care and Income: The Distributional Impacts of Medicaid and Medicare Nationally and in the State of Michigan,*

Dept. of Social Services, State of Michigan, Lansing, Research Paper No. 5, April 1971.

21. K. Davis, "Equal Treatment and Unequal Benefits: The Medicare Program," *Milbank Memorial Fund Quarterly,* 1975, 53:4, 449-488.

22. R. M. Bailey, "An Economist's View of the Health Services Industry," *Inquiry,* 1969, 6:1, 3-18.

23. R. M. Barkin, "Need for Statutory Review of the Health Services Industry," *Inquiry,* 1969, 6:1, 3-18. R. Roemer, "Social Regulation of Health Manpower," in *Fostering the Growing Need to Learn,* Division of Regional Medical Programs, Bureau of Health Resources Development, PHS, DHEW, Rockville, Maryland, 1974.

24. Citizens Advisory Committee on Environmental Quality, "Citizens Make the Difference: Case Studies of Environmental Action," Washington, D.C., Jan. 1973. N. Milio, *Promoting Health Through Public Policy,"* Philadelphia, PA, Davis, 1980.

25. G. A. Silver, "The Community Medicine Specialist: Britain Mandates Health Services Reorganization," *New England Journal of Medicine,* 1972, 287-25, 1299-1301.

26. J. Hastings, *The Community Health Center in Canada,* Ottawa, Information Canada, 1972. H. L. Laframboise, "Health Policy: Breaking the Problem Down into More Manageable Segments," *Canadian Medical Association Journal,* 1973, 108, 388-393. J. T. McLeod, "Consumer Participation, Regulation of the Professions, Decentralization of Health Services," a report submitted to the Minister of Public Health, Saskatchewan, J. T. McLeod Research Associates, Ltd., Regina, Aug. 1973. *Report of the Commission of Inquiry on Health and Social Welfare,* Government of Quebec, Vols. 1-7, 1967-1972. Quebec Province Bill 65, "Act Respecting Health Services and Social Services," 1971.

27. *American Behavioral Scientist,* 1971, September/October 15, Issue on Consumer Input. J. L. Falkson, "An Evaluation of Alternative Models of Citizen Participation in Urban Bureaucracy," Program in Health Planning, School of Public Health, University of Michigan, 1971. C. B. Galiher, J. Needleman, and A. J. Rolfe, "Consumer Participation," *HSHMA Health Reports,* 1971, 86:2, 99-106. A. W. Parker, "The Consumer as Policy Maker: Issues of Training," *American Journal of Public Health,* 1970, 60:11, 2139-2153. B. B. Wells, "Role of the Consumer in Regional Medical Programs," *American Journal of Public Health,* 1970, 60:11, 2133-2138.

28. J. D. Carroll, "Participatory Technology," *Science,* 1971, 171, Feb. 19, 647-683. L. S. Chapman, "The Neighborhood Health Center Foundation for Health Care: A Portent for the Future or a Necessity for Survival?" *American Journal of Public Health,* 1973, 63:10, 841-845. M. A. Costa, "An Interview," *Journal of Black Health,* 1974, 1:3, 24-29. *Public Administration Review (PAR),* "Symposium on Neighborhoods and Citizen Involvement," 1972, 22:3, 189-231. Society for Public Health Education (SOPHE), "Consumer Participation in Health Planning," *Health Education Monographs,* No. 32, 1972, San Francisco.

29. M. Olson, *The Logic of Collective Action,* Cambridge, Harvard University Press, 1965. *Citizens and Health Care,* B. Checkoway (Ed.), New York, Pergamon Press, 1981.

30. L. Meisner, et al., "A Training Program for Consumers in Policy-Making Roles in Health Care Projects," 1970, May, Continuing Education in Health Sciences, University Extension, University of California, Berkeley.

31. AACHP (American Association for Comprehensive Health Planning), "Consumer Participation Resolution," memorandum, Dec. 17, 1973.

32. M. M. Webber, "Alternative Styles for Citizen Participation in Transport Planning," Working Paper No. 143, January 1971, Institute of Urban and Regional Planning, University of California, Berkeley.

33. B. Daniels and C. Morris, "A View of Patients," *Journal of Black Health,* 1974, 1:3, 10-15.

34. California Supreme Court, "Court Sets Consent Guidelines," *American Medical News,* 1972, 15:50, 1-3. W. Gaylin, "The Patient's Bill of Rights," *Saturday Review,* March 1973, 22.

35. Ibid, No. 9. D. Mechanic, ibid, No. 19.

36. Ibid, No. 3. Ibid, No. 10. B. N. Shenkin and D. C. Warner, "Giving the Patient His Medical Record: A Proposal to Improve the System," *New England Journal of Medicine,* 1973, 289-13, 688-692.

37. Ibid, No. 10. J. Powles, "On the Limitations of Modern Medicine," *Science, Medicine and Man,* 1983, 1, 1-30.

38. Socioeconomic Report, *CMA,* XXI:7, Oct./Nov. 1981. D. A. McNutt, "GMENAC: Its Manpower Forecasting Framework," *American Journal of Public Health,* 1981, 71:10, 1116-1124.

39. "Directory of State Human Service Agencies," *Human Services Institute,* Washington, D.C., July 1974.

40. D. P. Andrulis and N. A. Mazade, "Mental Health Policy: Changing Administration and Directions from the 70's to the 80's," paper presented at APHA Annual Meeting, Los Angeles, California, Nov. 31, 1981.

41. R. Morris, ibid, No. 1.

42. R. Gumbiner, "FHP Pioneers Delivery of HMO Psychiatric Care," *FHP News,* Fall 1974, Family Health Plan, Long Beach, California.

43. I. Illich, *Celebration of Awareness: A Call for Institutional Revolution,* Garden City, Doubleday, 1971.

44. Ibid, No. 43. I. Illich, *Deschooling Society,* New York, Harper and Row, 1970.

Chapter 6

ATTRIBUTES AND TRAINING OF THE PROFESSIONALS WORKING IN THE PRIMARY CARE SETTING

In this chapter, we continue the fleshing out of our perceived needs, the **skills** called for in improving our health (**Box E** in **Figure 1.1**).

From what has been described as the appropriate workings of primary care, some deductions can be made about the attributes and the training of those who provide care for people and of those who carry out the related administrative and goal-support activities at the PWC. It should be clear that these prescriptions do not contemplate the disappearance of the "scientific" physician by the end of the century, as some postulate.[1]

I. CAPACITIES AND TRAINING OF THOSE WHO PROVIDE PRIMARY PERSONAL HEALTH SERVICES: PHYSICIANS AS AN EXAMPLE

We will begin by discussing the qualifications of primary care physicians, because they are presently the prototypical healers with the most independence and the most influence over care, and are the most needed of all physician categories.

Capacities I believe it is imperative that physicians have good grounding in the fundamental characteristics of all levels of systems. Their traditionally lopsided concentration on the somatic sub-systems of the person is clearly inadequate if health is heavily determined by the supra-systems of *homo sapiens.* Physicians need to be thoroughly familiar with the systems view of *homo sapiens* if they are to participate in caring for people, many of whose illnesses are likely to be social and psychic in origin, even though presenting in somatic or psychic forms.[2] They also have to have a concern for wellness. And if they are not personally interested in pursuing the strengthening of a client's health, or the well part of that person's life in the presence of illness, at least they must be sympathetic to health-promoting goals and to cooperate with those members of the PWC staff whose work includes the promotion of well-being. Above all they must have at least appreciation for if not skills of epidemiology in order to put into focus the health needs of populations, and thus of individuals in that population.[3]

Moreover, doctors who are trained in **averages**, and in normal distributions of a few somatic systems, must be made aware of the uniqueness of individuals, and the importance of individuals having the interest and capacity to participate in, if not orchestrating, much of their own care and in negotiating the caring decisions about themselves.[4] Also of importance is the physician's appreciation of the roles subscribers must play in the governance and planning of health care delivery if it is to meet needs, avoid foolish demands for care, and minimize pressure on servers, stemming from promotion of health behavior, self-help, and participation in providing the general care needs of the community. Physicians plead for patients to be more self-sufficient, yet with their obliviousness to the opportunities for patient self-help and participation in care they keep patients or consumers helpless at the door of the healers, whose paralyzing mystique pervades so many of their transactions.

Recruitment and selection Future primary care practitioners will have to be distributed in accordance with where the need for them is greatest. Mandatory years of service in specified locations is not going to be enough.[5] Distribution requires a system in which practitioners not only can work and make a living but are able to obtain needed services for their clients, have the opportunity for constant personal professional updating, and the opportunity for reasonable free time and relief.[6] It also requires recruitment and selection of persons with requisite capabilities and interest in primary care, and with an affinity for working in those areas which tend to be underserved.[7] Selection must then include a sufficiency of trainees to serve the unserved rural areas which exist in most of our 50 states, and the poorly-served, disadvantaged urban people, who are often a minority group as well.

In addition to selection, which requires more than concern for the community in which a candidate grew up, and selection in part by that community, which does help, and race, which does not always help,[8] and education in the area concerned,[9] a system of rewards and constraints undoubtedly will have to be engineered.[10] The incentives may have to operate directly on medical schools, so that they feel compelled to recruit and train selectively. Incentives directed at medical students, such as forgiveness of educational loans, have not worked too well. Legislation has been considered which uses more sophisticated incentives as well as mandatory location.[11] Its threat has been very effective in changing outlooks in medical schools.

It seems clear that if there were HCDS or MCDS delivery systems such as we describe, it would take a modest application of ingenuity to select candidates and have them place themselves in the poorly served areas upon completion of their training. In fact, many evident changes in the outlooks of new applicants for medical school suggest that it will become easier to recruit primary care physicians and get them to underserved areas (if incentives are so directed).[12]

Training Medical schools and most health professional schools get the pick of nimble minds, and probably a reasonable spread of dispositions and social attitudes. Our concern here is with the one-third of medical graduates (a higher proportion over the next ten years, in order to make up for current shortages) who are needed to be primary or family care experts. However, we see no reason for any physician to be deprived of what he or she most needs to understand—the origins and nature of health and its distribution in populations. Thus, the medical school training for all physicians needs the relatively new inputs which this book has proposed under the rubric of a systems view.[13]

Perhaps the most critical of all ingredients for training successful primary care practitioners is the step-wise ascertainment of their humanistic and technical competencies. Length of servitude, number of completed courses, and number of patients served do not provide reasonable assurance of competency.[14] Ways of checking elements of performance can and have been designed; many more are needed. Actual observation of performance on clinical cases can and must be carried out so that how well students do a task always includes how well they relate to their patients, and is accepted as the determinant of the duration of their training.

Teaching by traditional building blocks Probably we can continue, in great part, the teaching and learning of system-by-system (or parts of systems), each presented by the discipline most associated with it. We accept the limitation that this teaching tends to cross few system boundaries, crossings limited primarily to the systems directly above and below the area of central concern. But the best way to learn the fundamentals still may be by going into the necessary depth on each subject. Such teaching may go on in the laboratory, classroom, seminar, clinic, and wards, much as it does now. Hopefully, the means of presenting materials will make better use of teaching techniques that allow individuals to progress in their own way and at their own rate, matching their cognitive, analytic, and synthesizing skills with acceptable standards to test their progress. In this way when it is ascertained that students already know the material or can profit more from other modes of study they can avoid attendance at required courses and participation in every required activity in a given course.

Among the building blocks there is a critical need to include the social sciences and to cover such areas as sociological, economic, political, and administrative behavior, particularly as these relate to medical and health needs and care, general systems, and ecological outlooks.[15] As students are pressed to recognize the social implications of good and bad health for each of their clients, they must have an attractive and meaningful social-medicine curriculum into which they can dip for fundamentals.

Boundary crossing The general-systems approaches to patient care, decision making, planning, ecology, health, and other subjects that are based on boundary-crossing concepts, can also be taught, element by element, by the disciplines whose works represent special areas of boundary crossing. However, my limited experiences suggest that although most intellectually-agile persons can grasp the logic of boundary crossing, they still manage to compartmentalize their own attack on most issues to one or another system level depending on their dominant interests and skills, and on the facet which strikes them first or most forceably. The applications of boundary crossing in medical care do not necessarily follow from exposures and exercises available to a classroom. It is for this reason, among others, that clinical practice under appropriate supervision is so critical.

Clinical exposure Students usually crave the opportunity to assist directly with patient care, even at the initial stage of their professional development when they can barely guess at what is transpiring in the client or between the client and the doctor. Clinical exposure from the first day in medical school seems to be the best way to whet the students' appetite for acquiring the system-by-system fundamentals and relationships, which they soon come to realize that they must comprehend if they are to assist the person seeking help. Their interests in such basic disciplines as anatomy, physiology, psychology, social institutions, economic behavior, and so on, can rarely be captured so well as when they see the daily need to use these disciplines in behalf of individual clients. Under good clinical exposure to all supra- and sub-systems perturbations reflected in the requests and needs of clients, students do not have to be cajoled into studying what each discipline has to offer.

How the basic disciplines- and systems-levels content are taught probably matters minimally if boundary-crossing systems logic is joined continually with an understanding of the specific mechanics of each system level. Every client seen can provide a vivid demonstration of the interrelationship between systems when practitioner-teachers are capable of bringing this out by the means they use in relating to clients and unraveling their needs or malfunctions. Unfortunately, most of the medical students' present-day mentors themselves are aware of little more than physiologic and anatomic matters. If this initial student learning were to take place in the PWCs (with students following clients to secondary and tertiary care as needed), the disciplinary systems and ecologic approaches would soon be firmly melded in most students' minds. Those who find this person-oriented, mind-expanding experience too demanding can select a career in one of the disciplinary or super-specialized niches where a more-limited but highly-disciplined type of technical expertise is required.

What must be emphasized is that the students get their clinical training at the hands of primary care faculty.[16] Piecing together a wholistic and family outlook by rotating through secondary and tertiary care services under the tutelage of limited-system experts or, as is more customary, working on wards of the great medical centers populated with esoteric "cases" and presided over by disease-oriented experts, can only lead to an obfuscation of the needs of people for primary care. This is not meant to exclude a modest exposure of future primary care physicians to secondary and tertiary care. They must develop an appreciation of what goes on there and be prepared to use it wisely, as they safeguard the long-term best interests of their clients who occasionally need such care.[17] It has been well-stated that the three major values of training in a primary care center are **correction of the students' social ignorance, teaching them how to cope with uncertainty**, and **teaching them about the changing world of medical care.**[18]

Exposure to other skills and other resources Primary care experts must also learn the use of such other skills and resources as community diagnosis and analysis, and the use of social and psychic interventions. This means that their training must involve them with the persons with whom they will share client care in the PWCs. If they are denied regular work exposure to such persons in training, they may never comprehend their utility or undertake to work with them in practice.[19]

Faculty The big bottleneck to provision of suitable primary care clinical training is the current dearth of faculty who can illustrate the full caring and convening roles. The few who do it intuitively may or may not be seen as acceptable teachers by academia. The use of team teaching by available traditional health experts who do boundary-crossing may be the starting point. But present skills being what they are, they hardly illustrate primary care competency; rather, they illustrate an interest in it, and a fumbling (though good-hearted) attempt to create a new way of serving an individual. Perhaps we can also improve teaching of systems-oriented care by insisting that a single faculty practitioner be the designated convener for any given client. The clinical training experience we envision may also be enhanced by providing the assigned somatic faculty convener with both a psychic and a social level consultant, each intent on bringing out what is going on in their sphere of concern. As a team, they will search for the interventions needed at various systems levels for short- and long-term health improvements of a given client. And, as called for, they will incorporate in the overall client care what is obtained from other more-limited experts.

What has been proposed suggests new patterns of curriculum, and thus of faculty organization.[20] However, this does not mean that everything must be restructured. Horizontal natural and social science coordination, vertical preclinical and clinical coordination, organ system, functional team teaching, problem-based learning, and other cross-cut techniques may not be better than traditional building block methods in many areas. What is necessary is teaching the students from the patient, beginning on the first day at the medical school. This expands and slowly replaces subject-matter presentations to the point where it becomes the main mode of proceeding. By the second half of a students' medical education, disciplinary, organizational, or special-area presentations are superceded by clinical work to the point where the former become the occasional, but depth-adding, aspects of teaching. What is needed overall is new medical school leadership that has the care and health maintenance of people uppermost in their hierarchy of concerns.[21]

There is no point of going into the maze of residency training, except to indicate that the primary care physicians cannot settle for a tour of specialist services as their advanced training. They need to become proficient at boundary-crossing care, which is the essence of primary care. This will be acquired by being given increasing responsibility for primary care, under the tutelage of those very expert in this field.

II. CAPACITIES AND TRAINING OF THOSE WHO IDENTIFY AND ANALYZE COMMUNITY PROBLEMS, WHO PLAN AND DEVELOP PROGRAMS, WHO ADMINISTRATE, AND WHO ASSIST WITH COMMUNICATION

The major disciplines required For the purpose of this discussion, we will consider some of the major types of professionals trained by schools of public health: health educators, administrators, planners, maternal and child health workers, mental health workers, social workers, biostatisticians, epidemiologists, environmentalists, and so on. Of course, many of these workers receive comparable training in settings other than schools of public health nowadays. These professionals presently work mainly in the somatic and psychic service agencies, and the bulk of them do no laying-on-of-hands. A few, coming from one of such laying-on-of-hands disciplines as physicians or nurses, may continue to do some direct care in their original skill areas after taking on their new administrative roles even though their major work involves them in such activities as epidemiologic investigations, planning, designing, organizing, financing, administrating, and evaluating services and agencies.

The following is a brief review of some of the major disciplines currently being trained in public health schools, with suggestions for modifications in their capacities and duties if they are to relate to, or work in, primary care settings.

1. **Health educators** These are the communicators who will be needed in PWCs to help the various specialists understand and appreciate one another's work and to cooperate in the care of patients. Their major task, however, will probably be to bring about a participative relationship between the consumer and the provider, to encourage consumers to undertake more healthful behaviors, to get them to participate in processes which bring them systems thinking and survival wisdom, and to encourage and help prepare them for governance and planning body duties in the PWCs, HCDSs, and health authorities, where such exist.[22] These are important extensions of that vast field known as patient education.[23] If the health educators can extricate themselves from the position of "obtaining compliance," i.e., translating the professional's wishes to the consumer (rarely has the reverse been asked of them), they can put their general systems and behavioral background to excellent use in the new tasks outlined for them. For a more extensive discussion of the key roles to be undertaken by health educators see **Chapter 4.**

2. **Administrators** These are the connectors, facilitators, and task distributors who try to operationalize the policies of the PWC or HCDS. Their new jobs will be to integrate more and more disciplines into functional or purposeful primary care units rather than into disciplinary ones. The administrators will also have to link levels of organization, as between primary and secondary care. Their medical care expertise will have to be reoriented to that of health or well-being care. Their perception of the effects of systems on health will have to include health needs of populations and go well beyond the current orientation of most administrators to the mechanics of systems analysis and operations research in delivery systems.

3. **Maternal and child health (MCH) workers** These workers, who generally come from the ranks of obstetricians, pediatricians, and specially-trained nurses and social workers, will lose their sinecure in special-illness programs, but they may well become some of the most critically-needed PWC workers. They have the most legitimated access to

well people. Some of their well clients want children and some do not. Others are pregnant and come for careful supervision at a time of stress. Still others come for regular infant checkups and family supervision at a time of high risk. The MCH workers' ability to attract well people as regular clients can be capitalized upon to bring families of subscribers into the PWC for participation in its broader health-promoting activities.

4. **Mental health workers** These workers also have an opportunity to be center stage. Our perception of the psychic as being the key integrative aspect of the person-level system suggests that those most expert in this field are going to have the opportunity of being the major source of systems information. They assist with unraveling person-level blockages between supra-system and sub-system feedbacks, and of psychic relationships to social and somatic health. They should be of major help operationally in sorting out server and service malfunctions that block good patient participation and care in the PWC.

5. **Nutritionists** Because of the pervasiveness of food and drink in "fueling and lubricating" all bodily systems, these experts will play a larger role than heretofore. Systems logic indicates that more attention must be paid to problems of behavior and access in this area, for nutritional deficits have the capacity to cause unlimited perturbations by robbing systems of their reserves. Because much of the world's stability and individual well-being hinges on how wisely we use and share our food or food-producing resources, these workers will also be invaluable in helping with the survival-wisdom activities going on among the subscribers to the PWC.

6. **Environmentalists** These experts must also be present in each PWC to assist with the occupational problems to which subscribers are exposed. Also, they assist various groups, particularly infants, children, aged, and handicapped, who face high-risk environments. They use a combination of education about, and inspection of, client environments to improve the safety and quality of the physical environment. Their presence at the PWC enhances the likelihood that other servers will act on the environmental risks and dangerous behavioral patterns that are the major underlying causes of death and disability at younger ages. The environmentalists also will be invaluable in the survival-wisdom activities of the center.

7. **Social workers** These workers should have a field day in the PWC as the result of new insights about the social origins of psychic and somatic illnesses that will be gleaned from everyday caring, which goes on in an environment guided by general systems beliefs about health. They will have opportunities for experimentation and application of new interventions, with participation from many health servers and user-participants. Their role in disseminating survival wisdom can be a major one.

8. **Disease specialists** These workers, who will not be regular staff of PWCs, will be of help in situations where their area of expertise, such as diabetes, tuberculosis, venereal disease, or hypertension, is a particularly acute problem. However, they will have to move a long way towards systems understanding if they are to offer more than the dubiously relevant program suggestions typical of disease control activities in the past. When they are trained as epidemiologists or ecologists, they will make major inputs into the planning and evaluatory activities of PWCs and HCDSs.

9. **Basic disciplines** Experts in such areas as behavioral science, statistics, epidemiology, demography, or biology may not be full-time staff at PWCs, but they are going to have unprecedented opportunities for studies and experimentation with, and design of, new interventions as partners with HCDS staffs, subscribers, and boards. A good systems understanding of health not only suggests new ways of proceeding but opens up the whole world of existing data to re-investigation and re-interpretation.

Training How will this new comprehension of health and the boundary crossing that it requires be imparted to students in public health schools? To begin with, should schools continue to recruit and educate those who come with professional, health-relevant skills? Most professionals already cross a few systems levels and under the influence of boundary-crossing concepts, which will become a major emphasis at schools of public health, students should be able to break out of boundaries thrust upon them by prior training. From now on, more public health recruits will enter training with boundary-crossing outlooks that may well prod their teachers.

Can schools of public health continue to recruit many reasonably well educated, but biologically, scientifically, and systems-ignorant students for some roles such as administration and health education? Such students, who often are young and are seeking disciplinary or professional identification, come to schools of public health because they anticipate a career in which boundary crossing is taken for granted. If they don't find it being taught they are likely to be miffed. This outlook explains much of their enthusiasm for field work where they sense intuitively that all levels of systems confront and confound every human concern. Such students are generally enthused about tackling the complexity of reality, and enjoy unraveling the evidences of unsuspected forces that cause systems perturbations and ill-health.

Teaching by traditional building blocks What was said about physician training would seem to apply here, also: there is nothing wrong about teaching system-by-system or skill-by-skill, provided that modern techniques, built on performance testing, are employed for evaluation of learning. But, as in medical schools, there is a tragic weakness in social medicine, curricula, especially in such areas as policy formulation and economic and systems-type modelling.[25]

Boundary crossing What has been said about physician education applies here too: boundary-crossing concepts can be taught element-by-element.

Clinical exposure What is probably most effective in teaching, and accepted most enthusiastically by students, is the opportunity to analyze clinical situations which typically cross every level of system, and which use knowledge about each level of system. In most public health activities the clinical material consists of groups of people or communities who want relief from problems or assistance in reaching new levels of well-being. Sometimes the clinical material is a unit of government or an agency, such as a PWC or HCDS, created to render problem-solving assistance.

The average master's-degree-level students remain in school about 21 months, unless they come with already well-developed skills. The already skilled, as well as the novice, should get their first clinical exposure no later than the second quarter of training. The first few months are allowed for imparting such fundamental building blocks as statistics, computer science, economics, sociology, psychology, biology, health, and illness (whatever basic infrastructure the student is deficient in at entry). By starting a modest clinical exposure with a multidisciplinary group, preferably on the first day, several phenomena are likely to be encouraged. First, the students discover their ignorance of, and the need to master, the content of the very building-block courses which they otherwise barely tolerate and in which they often learn so little (typically statistics, epidemiology, and systems theory). Second, the field pressures on the students are transmitted to their instructors as pressures to make their courses more relevant to boundary-crossing perturbations that typify real-life problems. Third, boundary crossing becomes one of the most vivid and imperative dimensions of clinical work, and this is exactly what the successfully graduated practitioner will have to do. Finally, work with groups or organizations calls for inputs from many faculty. Students will have to pursue many sources of expertise other than those which can be provided by a single instructor or their classmates. This student-created incentive to cross boundaries and amalgamate disciplinary knowledge that comes from working on real-life problems is hard to resist.[26] My plea is that it not be resisted. Rather, it should be required that faculty participate in field teaching so that teachers enhance their own interdisciplinary, as well as disciplinary, skills by assisting students to assimilate building blocks in such a way that their contents are freely available and complementary, and make systems sense when applied.

Ideally, students will do their field work in small multidisciplinary teams which have a multifaculty seminar setting as home base. Here they present their findings, problem analyses, deductions, and synthesized proposals done for their team's client. The seminar faculty needs to include, as called for, the services not only of the substantive areas under consideration, i.e., maternal and child health (MCH), but the process experts. For example, if the student team is carrying out a planning or administrative task in MCH, there needs to be requisite planning and administrative faculty to consult in these process areas. For almost every team field situation, the faculty needs to include expertise on interpersonal relations and group behavior, for little gets done without human behavior being a major factor. Just getting the student team to work together may take a major *tour de force* by a well-qualified organizational and interpersonal behavior specialist.

Perhaps this suggests new patterns of faculty and curriculum organization. It certainly suggests the need for new ways of presenting knowledge in the basic science areas that students must master. There is no escape from the need for teaching towards objectives, and measuring performance accordingly. In particular, it calls for clinical experiences at the hands of a multidisciplinary faculty, although I doubt that team teaching is a routine necessity. Clinical exposure can be brief at first; but either it must be carried on part-time throughout enrollment or, alternatively, it must expand to nearly full-time for five to six months. This should be followed by a return to more-formal classroom exposures to skills or building blocks that the students, through their field experiences, have discovered that they need for development of expertise in their field.

The present-day typical field experiences in an agency, under the guidance of an agency or university-provided supervisor in the subject area that the students select for their career (or even the rotating experience of going from one specialist to another in an agency, or round of agencies), may find the students' learning all about boundaries but mostly how not to cross them. Their clinical work ideally should be related to the needs of a specific community or group. These are rarely covered by any one, or even by several, agencies. It is the doing of boundary crossing on behalf of clients with needs, assisted by the expertise called for from multiple types of faculty, student confreres, and practitioners, that should impart systems and boundary-crossing facility to the students by the time they complete their training.

The trainees' goals in the field are to render useful and desired services that fit with their needs for experience. They are not there to conduct studies, unless that is what is requested of them. They are also not there to do routine work which has no training value. This set of requirements probably calls for university-provided, competent, boundary-crossing, field work supervision.

Where the placement is in an agency, modest pay for the trainees strengthens the "relevant work" relationship desired. Where the placement is with a group or community, there may be no formal organization or funds. Here the tradeoff of useful work for experience must be emphasized. Under these stipulations, there will be no shortage of field placement opportunities. Every disadvantaged group is clamoring for help, every health planning body and every potential PWC and HCDs is seeking assistance.

Faculty incentives The typical university rewards system will need some turning around. Faculty in professional schools, in a general university, are often forced to slight teaching and minimize clinical work in communities in order to carry out research.

Research, which is regarded as imperative at such campuses, is most valued when it is **basic.** In practice, "basic" generally means research which is directed to creation of new knowledge for which the applications are not yet perceivable. In many universities, faculty are therefore urged to avoid **applied** research on community problems (applied usually means with the intent of problem solving). And overwhelmingly, it is so-called basic research and publication in refereed journals that determines tenure and promotion. Interestingly enough, the typical major argument favoring basic research is that some portion of it will find application some day.

Fortunately, some essentially free-standing public health schools, or those allied with medical schools, often have enough liberty to regulate their own reward systems. Some regard such quality clinical applications as teaching and applied research quite as highly as basic research, for use as criteria for faculty recognition and promotion. I will conclude with the thought that where solving human problems (applied research) is the object and subject of faculty and student activity, it would seem that inspiration for basic research should not lag far behind.

REFERENCES

1. J. S. Maxmen, "Goodbye, Dr. Welby," *Social Policy,* Nov./Dec. 1972, and Jan./Feb. 1973, 97-106.

2. G. L. Engel, "The Best and the Brightest: The Missing Dimension in Medical Education," *The Pharos,* 1973, October, 129-133. WHO, "Psychiatry and the General Practitioner," *WHO Chronicle,* 1974, 28, 65-70. M. S. M. Watts,

"Is It Time for a Fundamental Reexamination of Medical Education," Editorial, *The Western Journal of Medicine,* Nov. 1982, 137:5, 417-418.

3. J. R. Evans, "Measurement and Management in Medicine and Health Services," *The Rockefeller Foundation,* New York, 1981. *Community Oriented Primary Care,* Institute of Medicine, Washington, D.C. National Academy Press, 1982.

4. R. P. Biller, "Disaggregating Health Promotion and Health Care: Policy Initiatives that Depend Less on Homogeneity Assumptions and More on Human Uniqueness," Prepared for Conference On National Health Policy, February 12-13, 1976, San Francisco, Working Paper No. 49, Graduate School of Public Policy, University of California, Berkeley.

5. *American Medical News,* "Education Bill to Contain Shortage Area Service," 1974, August 19, 10. S. S. Wallack and S. E. Kretz, *Rural Medicine: Obstacles and Solutions for Self-Sufficiency,* Lexington, Mass., Lexington Books, 1981.

6. W. S. Beachem, "Appalachia, Testing Ground For Innovations," *Public Health Reports,* 1975, 90:4, 303-307. E. D. Martin, "The Federal Initiative in Rural Health," *Public Health Reports,* 1975, 90:4, 291-297. S. Wallack and S. Kretz, *Rural Medicine: Obstacles and Solutions for Self-Sufficiency,* Lexington, Mass., Lexington Books, 1981.

7. C. L. Hostetter and J. D. Felsen, "Multiple Variable Motivators Involved in the Recruitment of Physicians for the Indian Health Service," *Public Health Reports,* 1975, 90:4, 319-324. V. R. Neufeld and H. S. Barrows, "The McMaster Philosophy: An Approach to Medical Education," *Journal of Medical Education,* 1974, 99:11, 1040-1050. A. G. Rezler, "Attitude Changes During Medical School: A Review of the Literature," *Journal of Medical Education,* 1974, 49:11, 1023-1034.

8. M. A. Costa, "An Interview with M. A. Costa," *Journal of Black Health Perspectives,* 1974, 1:3, 24-29.

9. R. Kobernick, "WAMI, A Decentralized Medical Education Program in Washington, Alaska, Montana and Idaho," *Public Health Reports, 1975, 90:4, 308-312.*

10. D. Mechanic. *Politics, Medicine, and Social Sciences,* New York, John Wiley and Sons, 1974, Ch. 27, 271-278.

11. "Education Bill to Compel Shortage Area Service," *American Medical News,* 1974, August 19, 10.

12. J. R. Lave, L. B. Lave, and S. Leinhardt, "Medical Manpower Models: Need, Demand, Supply," *Inquiry,* 1975, 12:2, 97-125. I. S. Moscovice and R. A. Rosenblatt, "Rural Health Care Delivery Amidst Federal Retrenchment: Lessons From the Robert Wood Johnson Foundation's Rural Practice Project," *American Journal of Public Health,* 1982, 172:12, 1380-1385.

13. M. F. Hansen and K. G. Rich, "The Outline of a Curriculum," *Journal of Medical Education,* 1970, 45:1007-10. H. Rasmussen, Medical Education — Revolution or Reaction," *The Pharos,* April, 1975, 38:2, 53-59. J. R. Evans, ibid, No. 3.

14. R. A. Smith, "Towards Solving the Great Training Robbery," *The Pharos,* 1974, April, 47-52. D. Maddison, "A Medical School for the Future: The Newcastle Experiment," *World Health Forum,* 1980, 1:1,2, 133-138. R. E.

Ebert, "Can the Education of the Physician be Made More Rational?" *New England Journal of Medicine,* Nov. 26, 1981, 305:22, 1343-1346. B. Lo and S. A. Schroeder, "Frequency of Ethical Dilemmas in a Medical Inpatient Service," *Archives of Internal Medicine,* July 1981, 141, 1062-1064. C. J. Bland and D. G. Froberg, "A Systematic Approach to Faculty Development for Family Practice Faculty," *The Journal of Family Practice,* 1982, 14:3, 537-543.

15. R. Ebert, "The Program in Biosocial Medicine," *Harvard Medical Alumni Bulletin,* 1973, Nov./Dec., 20-25. H. H. Hiatt, "Healthy Thinking," Reported in the *Wall Street Journal,* 1974, Thursday, May 30, in "Politics and People."

16. R. J. Haggerty, "Graduate Physician Training in Primary Care," *Journal of Medical Education,* 1974, 49:9, 840-844.

17. Ibid, No. 15. J. Fry, *Medicine in 3 Societies,* New York: Elsevier, 1972, Ch. 2. 4-15. S. Jonas, "Some Thoughts on Primary Care: Problems in Implementation," *International Journal of Health Services,* 1973, 3:2, 177-187.

18. J. T. Hart, "Relation of Primary Care to Undergraduate Education," *Lancet,* 1973, Oct. 6, 778-780.

19. J. I. Bufford and D. Kindig, "The Next Two Years," Institute for Health Team Development, Montefiore Hospital and Medical Center, New York, 1974. H. B. Wise and D. Kindig, "A Planning Proposal," Institute for Health Team Development, Montefiore Hospital and Medical Center, New York, 1972.

20. J. J. Alpert and E. Charney, "The Education of Physicians for Primary Care," U.S. Department of HEW, Publication No. HRA 74-3113, 1973.

21. S. Jonas, ibid no. 17. V. Navarro, "From Public Health to Health of the Public," *American Journal of Public Health,* 1974, 64:6, 538-548.

22. H. S. Ross and P. R. Mico, *Theory and Practice in Health Education,* Palo Alto, Mayfield Publishing Co., 1981.

23. "Current Awareness in Patient Education," Department of Health and Human Resources, Center for Disease Control, Atlanta, GA, Sept. 1981, A Memorandum.

24. J. R. Evans, ibid, No. 3.

25. B. J. F. Mott, "The Future of Schools of Public Health," *American Journal of Public Health,* 1974, 64:4, 543-548. V. Navarro, ibid no. 21. E. H. Schein, *Professional Education: Some New Directions,* New York: McGraw-Hill, 1973. N. J. Stark, "The Future Health Administrator as Viewed by Others," in *Education for Health Administration,* Vol. 11, Ann Arbor: Health Administration Press, 1975.

26. T. Connelly Jr., R. Assell, and P. Peck, "Interdisciplinary Education for Health Sciences Students in the Rural Home Health Agency," *Public Health Reports,* 1975, 90:4, 325-330.

Chapter 7

A NATIONAL HEALTH POLICY THAT MOVES US TOWARD OUR GOALS

We, as a nation, must enter into a discussion of national health policy, with two understandings. The **first** is that we are in, and will probably remain in, an era of increasingly-limited resources.[1] The **second** is that individual health is affected more by environment and environmentally-induced behavior than by medical care. Yet, in the past 25 years we have allowed medical care to nearly double its proportionate consumption of our national resources while, by comparison, we continue to starve attempts to improve health-promoting, socio-economic, and physical environments for significant disadvantaged segments of our society, or to ignore the health effects of other major policies.[2]

Those of us concerned with health issues must also answer two basic questions: What portion of our wealth do we as a nation wish to devote to sickness care? and what portion do we wish to devote to improving health? Our proposals are for moving firmly in the new direction of emphasizing health improvements, rather than for more and more caring for health failures, including the preventable ones.

Sections **I** and **II** will present an analysis of our three major health issues, and examine the major alternative approaches generally available to achieve implementation (as applied specifically to the issue of cost control).

Section III presents the specifics of a national health policy that would enable us to overcome our three major failures (excessive cost, inequitable access to care, and poor health status). The policy is designed to bring us the **Institutions, Skills, Functions,** and **Processes** of care called for in **Chapters 4, 5** and **6,** so that they would "produce" better health, as described in **Chapter 2,** at reasonable cost and available to all.

I. THREE KEY ISSUES AND FIVE RELATED GOALS

It is possible to summarize the issues which focus everyone's attention on health and health care into three problem statements. It is equally feasible to summarize what we want done about them in five related goal statements as follows:

- **One problem is the unacceptably rapid, and apparently never-ending, increases in cost of medical care and in the proportion of national income spent for medical care.** *The corollary goal is effective cost control.*
- **A second problem is the inadequate and unfair distribution of health care services based more on the ability to pay for them than on the need for them.** *The corresponding second goal is effective equitable distribution of care.*
- **A third problem is an unacceptable level of health as exemplified by unbelievable variations from one place to another in our country, as well as our nation's very modest health status in comparison to other countries of the world.** *The corresponding third goal is the rectification of the poor health status of lower ranking communities and groups with an inordinately high risk of poor health.*
- *A fourth major goal* relates to and derives from the three prior issues and goals. *It is the redirection of our modes of delivering "medical" care, so that for the same or lesser levels of expenditure they become "health" care and make a more significant contribution to our health status.*
- *A fifth major goal is the wise utilization of the services we have, so that changes don't undo what we have that is good.*

An initial glance might leave one with the impression that satisfactory solutions to all of the three issues are incompatible. However, a more careful analysis of these three issues, and of the health/health care realities underlying them, will indicate that solving each of the three issues simultaneously is necessary in order for the solution of any of them to take place.

II. UNDERSTANDING HEALTH AND HEALTH CARE ISSUES

A. Escalating Costs of Health Care

Health care is an increasing proportion of the Gross National Product (GNP) The so called wealth-producing efforts of our country can be measured as GNP. There has been a continued increase in the GNP share taken by the health care sector. It was 4.6 percent in 1950, 5.2 percent in 1960, 8.3 percent in 1975, and 9.8 percent in 1981, when it took 287 billion. In 1983 it will be over 10 percent of the GNP.[3] The slackening overall economy suggests that health care will take an increasing fraction of our production, particularly if its costs continue to escalate as rapidly as they are now doing. The predictions of a slow economy for the next 20 years and beyond makes the trend even more ominous.[4] The public acceptance of such health care cost increases seems to be declining.[5]

Other sectors, and thus health, will suffer more as medical care takes a larger portion of GNP As we have seen in earlier chapters, health status is modestly affected by increasing amounts of medical care. On the other hand, health status is maximally responsive to general living conditions, and is particularly associated with level of education and with employment-income status. This suggests that the national efforts to improve health which would pay off the most would be directed to such constructive efforts as new or rehabilitated housing, low-energy mass transport, rebuilding deteriorating cities, and so on. These products not only help lower environmentally-induced psychosocial stress and physical hazards to health, but would create more jobs and more tax returns per dollar of expenditure than do the annual three to five percent real increases in health expenditures. Also, it should be pointed out that shifting resources towards "defense," from other services, removes perhaps 10,000 jobs per billion dollars of expenditure without leaving any useful or health-improving products for society.

1. Causes of the Increasing Costs

There are quite an array of forces affecting costs. We shall point up several major ones as well as list a large battery of probable or smaller ones. Basically, health sector costs are the product of units of service used and of the price per unit.

More people are using more units of care The increasing total national cost of health care reflects increases in use occasioned by such factors as: 1) growth in overall population; 2) growth of the aged portion of the population who need more care;[6] 3) increased accessibility for the traditionally less-well-served, through such redistributive devices as Medicare and Medicaid, or proposed National Health Insurance;[7] 4) presumed effects of better and more widespread general education and health education, which create awareness of untoward conditions as well as of the virtue of preventive and screening procedures; 5) increased technologic know-how, so that an increasing number of conditions are becoming amenable to intervention;[8] and 6) increased insuredness of consumers. These have two effects: general financial accessibility, and removal of significant pain on use of service.

There are two underlying features that suggest continued over-insuredness, 1) a genuine fear of financial risk from medical care;[9] and 2) the availability of employer-provided tax-exempt dollars that encourages expensive and redundant coverage[10] (even two insurance policies, when both spouses work), and the subsequent painless over-use of employer-provided insurance for benefits that are not worth their costs (the economists' "moral hazard").[11] Many question the importance of moral hazard and suspect that eliminating it may introduce dangerous "savings."[12] Evidence from other countries with mostly free care, such as Canada,[13] or Australia,[14] do not find the issue too impressive (but those are different societies).

In addition, there is the strong likelihood that unneeded units of work are promoted by a sizable underemployed segment of the more-autonomous health care professionals.[15] This force is in addition to the general incentives provided by a fee-for-service, non-risk sharing, professional approach to do more than is required, a reality which has been repeatedly documented.[16]

The skewing of rewards towards higher pay for specific procedures encourages specialization over generalist practice.[17] Yet many of these procedures may be of little value.[18] Related to this problem is the slowly-disappearing general practitioner and, in California, the declining medical student interest in family practice (including internists and pediatricians) which portends a continued decline, state-wide.[19] The relationship to costs may not be a small one, as the family practitioners probably see more cases per day, render more services per visit, and perform fewer fee-generating tests and procedures generally.

It is also worth emphasizing that we are still far from having created adequate access to care for all of our citizens and, if such were done, another significant source of demand would come into existence. In 1977 it was estimated that 18 million persons were totally without coverage, and that an additional 17 million were minimally or occasionally covered.[20] Moreover, not only was their use of services low but their health was poor.[21]

An even more discouraging aspect is the handling of the "frail dependent" as a medical case rather than as a social one, entailing specified medical services which are often needless,[22] and bundling the whole area into the health sector and onto its bill. A more complete listing of the causes of increased use of services is shown in **Box 7.1**.

Increasing price per unit of service and per case of illness There are a variety of forces at work which raise the cost and price of many units of service. Some are easily justified, others are not. Inflation is omnipresent but it is usually worse in the health care industry.[23] Such demand-raising programs as Medicare and Medicaid were not accompanied by any preplanned alterations in the distribution machinery. Underworked "autonomous" professionals, such as physicians, raise the price per unit of services

Box 7.1. Causes of Increased Use of Services

Demand-based Growth

- more per-capita income
- more government coverage
- more pain-free insurance coverage
- tax incentives for more coverage
- more medicalization of social needs, such as shifting aged from home to nursing home (avoids taint of welfare assistance and replaces role of extended family)
- more people
- more aging, more years of life, the sicker years
- more complex care leaving more seriously-disabled survivors
- more desire to use publicized, newly-discovered technology
- public ethos of keeping dear ones alive at any cost
- more education as source of more awareness and "want"
- new technologically-created accidents and diseases
- more urban residents = easier and cheaper access
- poor wait too long, then need more care
- rules and regulations force needless use of much care
- rules and regulations, and insurance, promote use of inappropriately-higher level of care when that is all they pay for
- many people still not covered, and offer a large reservoir of potential new users

Supply-based Growth

- new technological capacity that moves conditions into range of fixability
- new more expensive technology
- more specialization, dividing people up, more tests, more referrals
- fee for service—do more, earn more
- better payment and take-home for what is done in hospitals, so more is done there by doctors
- "cheaper by the dozen," so run dozens of tests (lab work skyrocketing)
- professional challenge to thwart death and do everything possible
- more iatrogenesis subsequent to all above
- different patterns of care in different areas
- quality controls push for highest denominator of procedures (PSRO algorithms)
- more physicians per capita, and less busy ones need to do more work to stay solvent (physicians generate 70 percent of health sector work)
- malpractice-induced defensive posture, involving more tests, records, etc.
- duplicatory services for different clientele in one area: as V.A. for eligibles, county for poor, usual private-profit and non-profit for others
- laws and regulations calling for minimum numbers of uses per piece of equipment
- continued shortage of generalists

to maintain their standard of living. Similarly, health facilities increase prices of their services which are underused. The open-ended, fee-for-service reimbursement for each unit of service, without any annually-negotiated prepayment for all of the care needed to cover a stipulated group of subscribers is probably the single gravest inducement to price increases. This not only induces more services, procedures, and hospitalizations, but removes concern with the cost of any one item, of any one episode of illness, or of the totality of care costs.

Relative Value Scales (RVS) also tend to set floors under charges. Payments by third party payors set above the mean, as is done by Medicare as well as other insurors, also are inflationary forces. Usual, Customary and Reasonable (UCR) fee scales also allow upward creep, even rapid upward escalation in communities where a few specialists dominate their specialty.[24]

More complex and more interesting are the inflationary effects caused by purchasers, such as Medicare and especially Medicaid, when they pay below real costs (also done by some Blue Cross contracts). This forces providers to resort to cross-subsidization, via higher-than-cost charges to those paying out-of-pocket or having more generous insurance. This situation not only raises the general level of charges but removes all incentives for providers to minimize costs.

The so-called empty-bed cost factor is no longer the "bugaboo" it once was. Beds not in use, particularly when they are in units withdrawn from service, probably add only a few percent to hospital costs: essentially debt service.

Another price-increasing factor is the substitution of higher cost technology which, although sometimes lowering the costs of care, is often more complex and thus raises costs in general. In the presence of shifting technology, Scitovsky and McCall point out that it becomes more sensible to count costs of care for a given condition.[25] In general, these have risen too. Moreover, new technologies open up opportunities for attempting heretofore impossible diagnoses and heretofore impossible therapies or support for the previously "hopeless" conditions. Overall, as much as 50 percent of the rise in hospital costs may be due to the use of new technologies.[26] **Box 7.2** displays a more extensive list of causes of price increases.

2. Means Presumably Available for Controlling Costs

There are primarily three: 1) use of **Regulation**, 2) dependence on the **Market**, and 3) the use of **Moral Suasion** and **Voluntary Effort**. We will examine the three approaches and look at their application to cost control. In this process, it will be seen that their role in our other two concerns, equity of access and improvement of health, are closely intermingled, and that some possible solutions for one are disasters for the others. On the other hand, some proposed solutions can be designed that help in the solution of all three problems of cost, equity, and health. The second half of this chapter lays out just such a set of solutions.

a. Regulation as Controller of Cost

Regulation is intended to serve many purposes. These may be listed as shown in **Box 7.3**.

In the sense that we speak of regulation, we refer to governmental agency activities to implement what is expressed in policies, laws, rules, regulations, and court decisions. This is done by such means as educating,

Box 7.2. Causes of Increased Price (per unit of service)

- general inflation
- health sector often "held up" on purchases
- many far-from-busy practitioners raise prices to maintain income
- many too busy practitioners raise prices to discourage access
- changing practitioners' life styles, with better hours, and less services, so charge more for services rendered
- excessively-rapid obsolescence of equipment
- shielding of consumers, doctors, and facilities from pain of financing by insurance and public programs
- tax incentives to buy more expensive programs: costs passed on to products and services
- overcoming historical under-payment of many classes of health workers
- fee-for-service professional and institutional payments
- relative value scales, which tend to set prices
- usual, customary, and reasonable approach to payment
- insurers (third party) have no incentives to control costs
- new techniques for doing a procedure are commonly better, but almost always more costly
- hospitals compete for doctors' patronage by equipping and building without regard to cost; winners have high costs, and losers higher ones
- over-building, with excessive overhead from unused capacity
- less philanthropy, and more borrowing with large interest costs by facilities
- costs of malpractice insurance
- multiple sources of payment, each with its own record forms and vying with the others to avoid paying
- many regulations add to accounting, sorting, hassling; just one CON procedure costs a "fortune" now
- threat of CON spurred a desperate flurry of acquisitions
- general systemic inefficiencies
- no risk sharing, so do work in most convenient, elaborate, expensive places
- no price-based competition, except for a few HMO saturated areas
- maldistribution of services, so that getting to them creates significant private costs
- maldistribution of services and incentives, causing use of expensive emergency rooms
- controls on independence of lesser-skilled and lower-priced health workers
- increased proportion of specialists who charge more for the same units of services
- transient gain and loss of eligibiligy to private as well as Medicaid coverage, with concomitant re-duplication of forms, tests, records, etc.
- shorter physician work hours and fewer patients seen per week
- free services provided by physicians are disappearing

funding, rewarding, supervising, policing, reviewing, holding hearings, prosecuting, and punishing. Coercion is the ultimate means by which government obtains compliance. It is used for purposes as different as obtaining a market or for replacing market activities.

1) Factors Facilitating the Successful Passage and Use of Regulation (Coercive Measures)

These factors can be summarized as follows:[27]

- The remedy will work
- The rule is consonant with market incentives to the maximum extent possible

Box 7.3. Nature of Regulation

- **Collecting taxes** Enables government to carry out its unavoidable collective affairs of governance, defense, education, and so on; this purpose facilitates all the others
- **Distributive** Gives something to many, e.g., Medicare, Medicaid. May have widespread but "hidden" redistributive aspects, when we consider who pays most and who receives most
- **Redistributive** Clearly undertakes to remove from one group or sector to provide to others; generally spoken of as removing from wealthy to help poor, as by income taxes; may take from poor and give to rich, as in redevelopment; may also take from one element of a sector (railroad) and give to another (trucking), as done directly by rate setting or indirectly by building highways; may take from some sectors and give to others (subsidies to agriculture, various industries, etc.)
- **Social regulation** Efforts at controlling dangerous environments (pollution), dangerous habits (driving helmets), appropriate creation of health services, review of Medicare and Medicaid charges, provision of informed consent, and so on
- **Economic regulation** Enforcing anti-trust laws (as would be necessary to prevent monopoly, or to improve function of the market)
- **Regulating natural monopolies** Where no market is reasonably feasible (water, power, sewage, and so on), total regulation is meant to act as a market substitute and to guarantee reasonable services at reasonable prices and profits. There is often a significant *redistributive* element here, as some consumers get services at less than the cost to serve them, while others pay more for the same product than it costs to provide it. This is also seen as a **substitutive** device to raising taxes, which would otherwise be necessary to pay for provision of essential services to a group that could not otherwise get them

Another way of viewing the functions of regulations is as follows:

- **Substantive** States the duties or requirements placed on those involved
- **Interpretive** States the meaning of legislation as applied to the situations under consideration
- **Procedural** States how the regulatory agency's activities are to be conducted, such as timing, hearings, and priorities
- **Guidelines** Provides an agency's advice to its clients on how to comply with a law or regulation; they may be recommendations or a form of moral suasion, where they do not have the force of law
- **Policy statement** Provides a sense of direction or intention, even though not in the form of Rules or Regulations; when a regulatory agency actually follows its policy statement by related actions, it may be accepted as R and R, and be so interpreted by courts

- The chosen remedy minimizes the cost burdens of compliance consistent with achieving the objective
- Benefits to consumers or to competition will substantially exceed the costs
- The remedy will not adversely affect competition, whenever feasible
- The remedy preserves or extends freedom of informed individual choice consistent with consumer welfare
- The remedy uses performance rather than input or process requirements, whenever feasible
- Only a few actors to coerce
- Citizenry want compliance widely and strongly (whether sensible or not), so that
  - enforcers do their job aggressively
  - enforcees make needed changes with minimal foot-dragging
- Few regulatory agencies involved
- Minimal ambiguity in policy, in what is wanted in way of process or product
- Good identifiability and measurability of what is wanted
- Available training and capacity among those who have to do the new job
- Size and clarity of penalties are high (and will be applied)
- Demand for banned product is low so that people will not pay a lot for bootlegged product
- General high respect for law and regulation in the society
- No one made to appear as a poor victim deserving sympathy, as a result of enforcement
- Violators not involved in key bargaining or power position

2) Regulatory Approaches Commonly Advocated or Utilized in Health Care Cost Control

Restraint of Utilization We are becoming accustomed to attempts at controlling utilization, even as we become increasingly aware of their failures. The extensive use of utilization review for Medicare, and increasing use of Professional Standards Review Organization (PSRO, P. L.92-603), reveals only extensive failures or minimal accomplishments.[28]

A variant of utilization control is the attempt to sort patients and direct them to proper levels of care. Already emerging, however, are suggestions that shifting patients to services of lesser capacities can mean prolongation of care, even patient regressions. At the same time, this approach may leave more-expensive beds empty while we try to create and fill less-expensive ones.

By itself, restraint of utilization by means of scrutinizing each health transaction when it is proposed, during its occurrence, or after its completion, represents the essence of expensive bureaucratic interference with the inevitable consumer incentives to seek, and provider incentives to prescribe, services whose costs are "hidden" by insurance, third party payers, and government programs. The likelihood of succeeding with such artifices remains slim, whether done by paid bureaucrats in an enforcing agency or by voluntary efforts of peer groups. Even if utilization controls could be made to work, producers could turn to price increases which neutralize the cost restraints intended by utilization-controlling legislation. In a report of a Conference on Quality Assurance in Hospitals,[29] there was little doubt about what a national group of experts meant when they said, *it is believed that with the current state-of-the-art in peer review, PSROs can generally detect and correct grossly inappropriate utilization of hospital services (which can produce some possible short-run cost savings), but it is doubtful that the PSRO program alone can have a significant impact on the rise in aggregate expenditures for hospital care. This view is based on a perception that these rises are due principally to factors beyond the control of the PSRO program.*

Price controls Price controls are cumbersome and essentially unworkable when restricted to a single sector of our economy.[30] Even among the fully-controlled utilities, there is little long-run evidence that price controls or rate setting has served to hold down prices. Moreover, in the health care field, increased or substitute provision of more-renumerative services is an effective counter to limiting costs by means of price control. If price control is pursued to the point of controlling procedures at the same time, it will lead to specified modes of care for most conditions; which is where the process orientation of PSRO quality activities is likely to lead, also. This is another hopeless patch, and one that in fact may escalate the use of needless but "required" services.

We may be led to think that arbitrary, below-cost, price ceilings, such as are typical of Medicaid, work, but experience tells us that they drive costs up for those patients not affected by ceilings. They also cause unwillingness and inability of the private sector to care for poor patients, who are therefore juggled back to expensive emergency rooms or to segregated facilities for the poor. This not only causes patient and record transfers, duplicated procedures, patient neglect, and confusion, but forces local government into maintaining a separate, inadequately-utilized system for the poor, which also becomes expensive as a result.

Medicare and Medicaid initially seduced the health industry nationwide, by means of cost-plus formulae, into reconstructing its facilities. But, now, these same programs are well along the road to enforcing below-cost price ceilings, which work devastating hardships on the very facilities which accepted the Federal "invitation" to replace and expand. These facilities have incurred a huge indebtedness as the result of borrowing, and servicing this debt accounts for a significant portion of hospital costs.

It must also be borne in mind that service costs can't be rolled back as long as hospitals survive by competing for physician patronage. Success means more of everything: more indebtedness, and higher costs for the winner. This means equally higher costs for the loser, which has to carry its unused facilities and services by increasing prices, and thus earnings, from those of its facilities and services which are being used.

Reviews of prospective rate setting hold more promise than retrospective methods[31] (see **lids**, page **164**).

Restraint of productive capacity This approach is dependent on the logic that if there are fewer providers, services, or facilities there will be less ability, as well as temptation, to provide unneeded services, and that those available will be used more adequately. We have already referred to the evidence that excess supply, or underutilized manpower or facilities, do promote increased units of work or increased prices if the providers are to survive.

Clearly, we will be seeking to restrain the rapidly-increasing numbers of providers in specialty fields which are now badly oversupplied.[32] Such attempts at control are now affecting medical schools in the form of removal of Federal training capitation-support funds. As a result, medical school fees are going up, and their applicants will shift further away from being members of underserved groups. However, there is no evidence that the total number of trainees will decline or that the rising practitioner-population ratio will be slowed.[33]

Other attempts to restrict productive capacity have been launched in the form of state Certificate of Need, and Federal Social Security legislation (Sec. 1122 of the Social Security Act, P. L.92-603), and the planning legislation, P. L.93-641. Since hospital care is the most costly and the fastest rising cost element in health care, it is thought that successful restriction of needless capacity would bring their operations to a higher percent of capacity. This should provide two economies: lower cost per unit of service, and removal of inducements to fill empty beds or provide needless services.

All the evidence on ability of these approaches to restrain development of new facilities and services successfully is dubious at best. In an extensive study, Lewin and Associates were unable to find convincing evidence for the value of such controls.[34] They are not alone.[35]

With the declining use of hospitalization, the acute general hospitals add technologic capacity rather than beds, and replace older beds even in the presence of over-bedding.

Lids Lids can be placed on monies available to any or all elements of the health care providers. The Carter Administration proposed such a cost control on hospitals. In general, the idea was to limit the total a hospital could earn in a year, based on prior performance. This would be irrespective of general inflation, new technology, changing patient mix or age, new clients, and so on. Naturally, this would prevent any shifts from one service element of the sector to another. It might even cause a shift of cases from more efficient to less efficient centers. It has been well-described as "fiscal strangulation," and blind at that.[36]

More sensible variations, such as prospective budget negotiations, can be carried out with HMOs (HCDSs) or hospitals as well.[37]

Varying piecemeal-lid approaches were the order of the day in 1981-82.[38]

The ultimate lid: a Congressionally-budgeted-and-financed single national pool of health sector funds Under this lid, the total national bill for health services will show up in one place at one time, as part of the national budget, prior to its expenditure. There will be no way that the cost of health care can creep up silently, as it does now, and become visible for the first time in the form of a year-end summation of where the dollars have gone. The costs for a given year will be evident a year in advance. They will be debated and set against nationally-voiced demands for housing, education, defense, transportation, and so on. Collectively, we can, for we will have to, face up to what we want, and call the shots accordingly. This is the most basic cost-control approach, for it limits or puts a lid on the total resources that can be raised and spent nationwide for health care. This approach collects in one place all of the funds to be used for the health care of rich and poor alike. (The monies can be raised by one or many Federal mechanisms, such as a) payroll- or social-security-type deductions, b) general funding heavily derived from income taxes, and c) special taxes.

These nationally-pooled funds must then be allocated to full service systems (HCDSs) on a prospectively negotiated, annual, full-coverage basis for all the health care of all their enrollees. (All persons will subscribe to one or another HCDS of their choice.) Regional differences in costs of producing services, and demographic differences of subscribers that call for more or less services, would enter into the allocations to each HCDS. What is important about putting all the funds for all of the services for a specific group into one fund are the opportunities it provides to give people the services they need at the levels called for, and the opportunities for the organization to make savings which it could share among producers and subscribers.

3) Problems with Regulations

There are numerous reasons why a coercive regulatory approach to health-care cost control in the U.S. has been both unpleasant and unsuccessful, generally. These are presented in **Box 7.4**. From a very practical standpoint, it is clear that we have had few tangible results on any score from CON or PSRO controls, while a few reports seem to indicate restraint on bed building.[39]

b. The Market as Controller of Cost

1) Nature of the Market and Competition[40]

The market can be briefly described as follows:

- It is a place of voluntary exchange
- Multiple similar and dissimilar producer goods provide consumer choices among products of a like nature, and among products with totally different utilities (health care versus recreation, for example)
- Profit-maximizing firms produce goods and services
- Utility-maximizing consumers pay for these goods and service out of their own income
- Within the framework set by market prices, firms control the cost and quality of their products, and their search for maximum profits leads them to minimize the costs of what they produce
- Because consumers pay for what they consume out of their own incomes, they are cost conscious and the prices they pay reflect their marginal valuations of the goods and services they buy
- If excess supply develops, competition forces market prices down
- As prices fall, less-efficient firms leave the industry, other firms may curtail production, and the excess supply eventually disappears
- On the other hand, if excess demand develops, prices are bid up, new firms enter the industry, other firms find it profitable to increase production, and the excess demand is eventually satisfied
- In competitive industries, market pressures discourage in-

Box 7.4. Reasons for Regulatory Failure

- **Conflicts between legislative intents** when subsequent regulations are carried out fully (anti-trust vs. health planning directives)
- **Regulations don't match their legislation**, and either distort, run counter to, or ignore legislative intent (has given rise to a whole new institution of public and legislative reviews of proposed regulations)
- **Regulations may concentrate on the wrong things** For example, they may focus on the easily-observed or measured which may be trivial relevant to the intended purpose; they may concentrate only on the large or the small operations, when the major concerns lie in the other; thus they do not achieve what is intended, they annoy those policed, they anger those to be protected, and they disgust the legislators
- **Regulations die hard** Constituencies are formed among: 1) those who are being protected or aided, 2) a large majority of those who are being regulated typically, since regulations can easily become a shield against change in an industry or sector, can provide subsidies, remove competition, guarantee profits, prevent new entrants to the field, even prevent new approaches to the same area from other sectors (energy, transport, communications), and so on, 3) those who make a living out of carrying out the regulations, and 4) those politicians and others who don't look forward to changes, or fear them; where such matters as unemployment in the ranks of those regulating or of those being regulated may result, meaningful changes are particularly hard to achieve
- **Regulations retard innovation** Many regulations dictate the nature of inputs, the process, the outputs, or their distribution, so that attempts to introduce significant change which many might want may be blocked in every direction
- **Cross-subsidization** often occurs as one type of regulation affects reimbursement *vis-a-vis* costs in an abnormal manner, so that as one service loses another that is uncontrolled must charge its customers more to make up for the loss; in this way, keeping track of "real" costs become enigmatic, irrational, and always unfair and wasteful
- **Externalities** of various sorts may be created or hidden; cross-subsidization is one example; another is keeping people in expensive hospital beds for lack of skilled nursing facility (SNF) beds, because Certificate of Need (CON) has been used to hold down the burgeoning state-level Medicaid cost by keeping down the numbers of SNF beds; another is the low physician fees for Medicaid, that find them turning patients to emergency rooms (ER) which will cost two to four times a customary physician fee
- **Destruction of a much needed but economically-weak product or producers** (ghetto-serving doctors or hospitals adversely affected by below cost reimbursement of Medicaid)
- **Decline in ethical standards** Unfair and unreasonable regulatory demands on health providers erode their feelings, voluntary support, and behavior, just as prohibition made providers into bootleggers and consumers into their law-breaking customers, so can provider and consumer be taught total disrespect for government authority; as a result, the corrosion of a supportive outlook towards regulation for what is good for society can, and probably has, spread to the integrity of dealings by provider and consumer in the health sector to a greater degree than we wish to tolerate, although perhaps not so far as in other sectors
- **Adverse political or attitudinal feelings about government, its programs and its regulations**
  - **on victims of conditions under consideration**
  - **on producers**
  - **on citizens, generally**
  - **on enforcers**
  - **on law makers**

Box 7.4. (continued)

- **Regulations may produce many costs, some hidden** In each of the cases above, there are obvious forces creating costs:
  - for government, in carrying out the regulation: for overcoming overlapping and disagreeing regulations; for preparing new legislation, hearings, studies, special procedures to control new legislation; to overcome avoidance tactics of enforcee, public distaste; or achieving resources to facilitate successful use of coercive measures, etc.
  - the actual costs of surveillance, tests, records, training, punishing, etc.
  - the costs to those regulated a) for **compliance** with the various procedures, records, data collection, reconciliations with regulators, and legal contests with regulators; this involves studies, structure and process changes, training, increased or decreased material and personnel costs, time for inspections; estimates range from two to 20 percent of hospital costs as being due to regulation (it is also true that many if not most of such costs would be incurred 1) if one ran a safe, well-managed show and cared to know what one is doing, such as keeping financial, production, and other records, planning, managing, and controlling that should be done by any industry that cares about its future, and 2) much of which would have to be done if it were in a competitive market); b) for **avoidance** of compliance in preparing injunctions, suits, lobbying, threatening, and advertising
- **Costs of regulation** ultimately fall on the consuming public, generally, but sometimes go mostly to those who do not stand to gain from the regulating
- **Costs of responding to regulation** may prevent needed change, or at least discourage consideration of change (foregone opportunity cost)
- It is still possible that the net gain to consumers or society overall, from conservation of resources, safety, prevention of needless procedures, etc., may far exceed costs

efficient production process and unwarranted, high-cost technology

- The nature and volume of choices struck up between buyers and sellers determine what is worth producing, i.e., this is **market authority** as described by Lindblom[41]

As Lindblom points up, the market can be found at work not only in capitalistic, for-profit centered economics; it has been intentionally introduced into communistic anti-profit economies, which have perceived that **market authority** may be to a great extent more relevant and infinitely less costly in driving the market than is **governmental authority**. **Governmental authority** is that in which legislators and bureaucrats reason out the nature, volume, and cost of what is to be produced, in accordance with politically-determined goals, consumer needs, diverse constituencies, and the inevitable resource constraints.

In recent times, the political right has also made the word "market" synonymous with the removal of all regulatory controls, or to the selective removal of controls which any one group of providers happens not to like or want. (We are seeing how medical providers, for example, literally abhor removal of controls and creation of a real market.) Of course, in order to ensure the reality of a meaningful competitive market there is a need for heavy, as well as carefully-thought out, regulation in order to avoid monopoly, cartels, and various competition-strangulating devices so dear to the heart of for-profit producers.

Requirements of the unfettered health market place These can be listed as follows:

- free entry of anyone into the ranks of producers
- Producers can make and sell any product, with any kind of labor, anywhere, for whatever price they can get
- No domination of price or exchange by large producers or large buyers
- Producers are price "takers," not "setters"
- Producers are at risk for their investments, contracts, sales, profits, survival
- Buyers are free to buy any kind of product at the best price they can achieve, without insulation from such financial pressures by insurance, or income tax exemptions for health care or insurance costs
- Good, easily available information on all services, costs, etc.
- Ample consumer choice as to product, price, and producer

It takes strong coercive regulation (as anti-trust) and firm policing to make sure that there is no collusion among sellers or among buyers to avoid the risks offered by the "pure" competitive market place. In fact, health care seems like a particularly-unsuitable sector to perform reasonably in a heavy market atmosphere, given the **GOALS** it is expected to reach, the history of its development, and consumer-provider relationships over a set of products which is hard to describe or price. The latter factor is one reason that relatively-complete service packages, such as "full" care by an HCDS (HMO) for a full year (not unlike a whole automobile), can be priced; and only then can health care services be competitively marketed for price.

It should also be noted that health care insurance, *per se,* is also considered to be a classic example of market failure because it inserts moral hazard, i.e., consumers can painlessly spend the insurers' money on so-called benefits not worth their costs.[42]

2) Types of market approaches that have been suggested or tried

Individual, consumer-set health care consumption priorities (i.e., no more health insurance and no more moral hazard) An approach that will reduce demand or consumption, and thus probably affect total costs, is to return to the individual consumer the payment, and thus the pain, of making decisions about what to spend **his** or **her** money for. There is little doubt that removal of insurance, or off-setting it by requiring large up-front deductibles, or continuing out-of-pocket patient payments, such as a significant percent of co-insurance or specified amounts of co-payments, will cut usage.[43] This must be rejected as being basically inequitable for it penalizes the poor, unless it has a built-in sliding scale of out-of-pocket charges based on income. It probably also inhibits use of health promotive or preventive care, and increases use of hospitalization as a consequence of neglect.[44]

A modification of this approach is to remove the income-tax sheltering that the average employed person receives on an employer-paid health policy. Many proposed schemes include total abandonment of such tax sheltering, fixed ceilings on employer contributions, cash rebates for employees who select less-costly plans, as well as heavy reliance on larger deductibles, co-payments, or co-insurance. There is reasonable agreement about the efficacy of the latter devices.[45]

Is this approach of putting the pain and the personal economic control back onto each family even conceivable in the U.S.? Possibly so. But hard-won, tax-exempt, fringe-benefit health insurance, with modest or little co-payment, is a big take-home item for perhaps 50 percent of our families. Moreover, there is ample evidence that most people tend to over-insure in this area, wanting no risk whatever. They buy supplemental coverage even when redundant, as is well exemplified now in the multiple insurance coverages bought to cover Medicare gaps.

Group competitive insurance This approach was popularized by Ellwood, and more recently built into a more-encompassing policy framework by Enthoven.[46] Such competitive proposals generally build in one or more of the following features:

- Providers organize into competing economic units capable of offering a complete set of services for a fixed price, for each subscriber, for a period of a year
- Providers are at risk for fulfilling the contractual agreements at the price taken
- Each worker (subscriber) has a choice among several plans offered at different prices
- All plans have identical basic coverage and must observe the same basic rules, but costs vary primarily according to differences in levels of deductibles or co-payments and, in some cases, in accordance with special-benefit features
- Congress will set a limit or cap on, or eliminate entirely, the tax exclusion on employer funds provided for health insurance of employees
- Employers must pay the same amount towards any plan they offer, and where the employee-selected plan is less expensive

there is a cash rebate to the employee (it need not be the full amount)

- Low-income persons receive vouchers from the Federal government with which to purchase membership in a plan

The assumptions about, and defects of, such plans are vigorously debated. The forces arrayed against such proposals are said to be formidable.[47] The major protagonist points out that, like all market-based schemes, they must be guided by stern and well-thought-through regulation. If not, the disasters that struck the Prepaid Health Plans (PHPs) of Medicaid in California are going to be relived.[48]

A whole new array of so called price-cutting and discounting efforts are being put in place. Most depend on heavy utilization controls (which obviously never work) to insure that providers do not perform more units of service to make up for lowered unit of service prices. These gimmicky so-called competitive approaches were given a firm boost by AB3480, passed by the 1982 California legislature. Many descriptions, prognostications and fears have been expressed about them.[49] In my opinion the main benefits of trying such approaches are not the dubious health care cost savings but the nudge they are giving to large employers and insurors to participate in the health sector's health. In turn, their concerns are creating a much more receptive health care industry response to health sector finance concerns.

Enforcement of anti-trust or anti-monopoly behavior, so that the health sector is more nearly on a market basis Havighurst is the best-know exponent of this line of reasoning.[50] He points up the many things that can be done to bring us to a more realistically-performing market. These are primarily:

- remove restrictions on professional advertising
- prevent the price fixing inherent in such measures as Relative Value Scale (RVS) and Usual Customary and Reasonable (UCR)
- remove professional or institutional control of such entities as Blue Shield and Blue Cross
- ensure more open entrance to the professions, and of more professions to practice both in and out of institutions
- allow all reasonable forms of provider organizations, corporations, etc. to enter the field
- prevent professional boycotts and restraints of trade, and allow collective bargaining
- remove professional "prescriptions" as to how professionals are to be employed, paid, and so on

- remove professional restrictions on contract practice

Costello points up the need to give market competition a chance by utilizing firm anti-trust action against private interference with the medical marketplace.[51] On June 15, 1981, the Supreme Court made it clear that devices used to exclude competition would not stand up under anti-trust legislation. However, because the case heard was a murky one for other reasons, it is not clear whether planning done under public auspices, such as P. L.93-641, could indeed limit competition.[52]

3) Market failures

These are so extensive and so critical in the health sector that they bear relisting. In essence, they represent the major reasons already presented for justifying governmental intervention. Nationally, the market's major failures are: 1) its inability to reach highly-valued societal goals, and 2) its inability to maintain itself without continued government intervention. The very definition of property, which varies from legal system to legal system, defines what the market is all about in a given country at a given time. The market is a total artifact of property law, and thus can be, and is, being changed constantly by new laws, i.e., there is no God-given formula for the market nor guarantees of its virtues. It is changed by laws establishing rewards, tasks, and so on.

It seems safe to say that pure market "authority" cannot be expected to achieve much of any of our highly-held **GOALS** shown in **Box 7.5.** (The **GOALS** are not entirely separable; they overlap and constrain one another in many ways: going to an extreme on any one may seriously limit others). (See **Regulation**, pages **159-65**, which are set up in part to overcome market failures in achieving a society's fundamental goals.)

It is probably true that all of these types of market failure are manifestations of what are described as "externalities." These are the benefits or costs not capturable by, or collectible from, the producer. Most impressive are the negative externalities, such as air pollution, where all neighbors pay for the damages while the producer of the pollution keeps production costs down.[54]

In concluding our observations on the market, it must be noted that it is not the only source of competitive efforts. What is very evident today is the almost cut-throat competiton among non-profit, as well as for-profit, hospitals that has been unleased by various reimbursement lids and caps placed on these providers. It is also important to observe the reluctance with which the violently anti-regulatory American Medical Association (AMA) is approaching anything that might resemble a real market.

c. Voluntary Effort (VE) and Moral Suasion (MS) in Cost Control

1) Nature of VE and MS

Both **VE** and **MS** are highly related in the sense of being guided by ideals and aspirations that are neither direct responses to traditional profit motivations nor government command. **VE** and **MS** have much in common. **Moral suasion** speaks to inculcating the devotion to valued standards of behavior (moral), and the ability of one or another institution to persuade (suasion) others to accept the moral tone and act accordingly, without promise of profit or threat of penalty. **Voluntary effort** represents behavior that creates institutions to carry out certain activities (generally intended to be benevolent or to facilitate some "higher" purpose) which

Box 7.5. GOALS

- **Fairness** In the health sector, this includes equity of financial and geographic access to care irrespective of means and, particularly, assistance to the disadvantaged. It typically implies significant redistribution of wealth and opportunities which the market cannot do; obviously, many rural, and all poor, communities will get little from the market
- **Keep the market open** Providers now work hard to exclude entry, prevent new kinds of competitive arrangements, set product standards and prices, work hard to foster government-sponsored demand for services and guaranteed higher recompense, minimize availability of meaningful information to consumers, and so on [53]
- **Improvement of health** This includes maintaining quality and safety of care, and promotion of prevention. The market will probably not produce much of prevention since individuals are not prepared to pay for that, preferentially; nor need the market concern itself with quality or safety, for it may find it cheaper to pay occasional damages than to make a safe product (the auto industry); and consumer knowledge can only be too little and too late, particularly for medical services
- **Public protection** This includes public safety measures, such as non-flammable night clothes for children, police and fire services, safety of workplaces, air, water, food, and sewage disposal. Individuals cannot be guaranteed these by the market; they are attainable only by protective regulations and measures control
- **Reasonable level of total costs of health sector** The market has little to do with sectoral cost limits; it may expand the sector almost endlessly until competition between sectors becomes effective. Notwithstanding, any one sector may be so effective or attractive, market-wise, that it grows to the point of being overwhelmingly societally-harmful, unless restrained (steel-auto-gasoline-highway axis prior to the late seventies)
- **Market process also means squeezing out the "inefficient" producers,** so that only a few producers are left (whereby competition disappears). To keep from getting such a market-produced oligopoly, or even a monopoly, government has to step in to split up companies, provide subsidies, create tariffs, etc., so that the less efficient can survive and maintain the illusion of market competition. Thus we need a non-market government force to maintain a semblance of market, even one that can never be much of a "free" market anyhow
- **Markets pay no attention to conservation of scarce resources,** and may even hasten their exploitation and destruction at times of long-term shortages. The boom-and-bust cycles which result from market expansion and contractions are also terribly wasteful of human, as well as natural and man-made, resources (abandonment of Detroit and other central cities)

assists others, whether as individuals, groups, or governments. They may spring up *de novo* or in response to **moral suasion** from any source.

In either case, it must be recognized that much of the behavior induced by **MS** or **VE** may be indirectly stimulated 1) by hoped for profits as spin-off from the good image earned by the behavior, or 2) by a perceived threat from various quarters if it is not undertaken. (See **Boxes 7.6** and **7.7.**)

2) Roles Assigned to VE and MS

In my opinion, the outstanding importance of the voluntary sector generally is ignored, in spite of the huge role it has played in most democratic societies; even in those which seem to use it the most effectively.[57] Its role in health care alone entitles it to more serious consideration.

Recent attempts to utilize VE and MS The AHA has promoted **VE** nationwide in an admitted attempt to avoid a renewed imposition of the Nixon-initiated price freeze, and to delay any far-reaching new regula-

Box 7.6. The Nature of Moral Suasion

- It puts the initiative for doing a prescribed type or scope of behavior directly on the individual or institution, by means of creating conviction rather than depending on profit or punishment to enforce the behavior
- Whether **MS** is created effectively by government or other groups, strong support can be roused for individual or institutional behavior, as varied as desiring or participating in markets or in desiring and complying with regulations
- It depends on a valued sense of direction or guides that have been internalized as being terribly important
- The uniformity of these internal guides, across the population groups concerned, determines the effective level of **MS**
- It provides a "conscience" against which one checks one's own behavior and that of others

The sources and use of **MS** appear to be about as follows:

- Each society instills internalized guides as well as the degree of vigor with which one should pursue desired ends and make demands of others to do likewise
- Social groups and associations may do likewise intentionally, educating, reinforcing, rewarding, punishing;[55] they may work at cross-purposes to the larger society or culture, or in new ways (**VE** in health sector in the U.S.)
- Government may do likewise intentionally, using education, rewards, punishment, etc.; it may rule more through such devices than through tangible planning, jiggered markets, or coercive regulation[56]
- Governments can go only so far in coercive regulating or in enforcing markets, unless people are morally suaded to go along to new levels; even the most-successfully repressive society comes to the breaking point; therefore, governments which mean to move drastically in new directions have to do a tremendous job of moral suasion, or face being challenged
- Use of **MS** may be accompanied by many rewards or threats, to get attention and a hearing

tions.[58] The effort appeared to be working well during the period when the hospital industry inevitably plateaued in the seventies from its frantic Medicare/Medicaid-induced building efforts of the late sixties. But, beginning in the late seventies, new and replacement needs in both technology and facilities, combined with the below-cost reimbursement tactics of government programs, especially Medicaid, forced new rounds of rate increases. By 1982, hospitals again reached some of the highest annual rate increases ever.

Renewed efforts In California, the California Voluntary Effort (CVE), sponsored by the California Hospital Association, the United Hospital Association, the California Medical Association, and many

Box 7.7. The Nature of Voluntary Efforts is Somewhat Different Than MS

- It allows a group of individual persons or institutions voluntarily to create new institutions, relationships, or a set of postures to create what:
  a) the individual could not do singly
  b) the government or society is too poor to create, given other pressing needs
  c) government will not be allowed to tax for, because a majority of people are:
    1) not aware of the existence of a need, e.g. hospice
    2) not convinced of the value of certain services, e.g. a center for independent living for the disabled
    3) opposed to taxing the many for the benefit of a particular group, or for servicing a given condition
    4) opposed or not accepting of a service because of esthetic, religious, philosophic, or ecologic beliefs (Planned Parenthood prior to the sixties)
- When the larger society has been won over by the outcomes or good work of the **VE**, society is likely to take on the entire activity for all persons
- It allows avoidance of the fears attached to the "unscrupulousness" of the proprietary or for-profit market activities, in such areas as hospitals, rehabilitation centers, etc.
- It allows avoidance of the stigmas of government services
- It allows avoidance of the fears of extension or growth of government, whether for reasons of control or efficiency
- Some **VE**s give the impression that they share the entrepreneurial gifts of the market, and the impartiality and accountability of government
- Some **VE**s give the impression that they share the inertia of government, as well as the public unaccountability of private enterprise

The sources and uses of **VE** can be summed up as follows:

- Many countries actively support **VE**s by removing taxation, even by outright grants, thus avoiding the need for government itself to create the institutions or services even when they are widely desired, respected, and willingly funded from taxes
- Many countries support **VE**s because they want a non-government, private, nonprofit way of providing the goods and services its people want; the degree to which this is done may vary from sector to sector in one country
- Many countries support **VE** because of desirability of lower taxes, as a result of religious, benevolent, fraternal, and philanthropic organizations providing financial support for hospitals, rest homes, hospices, schools, visiting nurses, blood banks, old age payments, and so on

business, labor, and even state agencies, went into action on a very broad front in the early eighties. These included advocacy of an array of interventions to exercise restraint on new ways of delivering care.[59] They even tried to breathe life back into such a "dead horse" effort as **utilization review,**[60] which suggests an attempt to buy time from more stringent regulation, or lids, or open price competition. (It died in 1983.)

3) Failures of VE and MS

These include some demonstrated and hypothetical bad outcomes, which are listed in **Box 7.8.**

d. A Spectrum of Choices to Implement Cost Control

Figure 7.1 presents a view of the interrelationships of how the three major modes of obtaining policy implementation, just described, can and do interact. Of course, what is indicated here is applicable to the implementation of all social changes or purposes, not just to those of cost control in the health sector.

The individual as the originator of choices among the options Individuals (**Box A, Figure 7.1**) are seen as desiring certain **GOALS,** which only can be attained: 1) by collective organized action, for which they require a formal governance structure (**Box B**); 2) by individual strivings which proceed satisfactorily in a "pure competitive" market (**Box C**), limited only by the constraints of the **GOALS** requiring collective action; and 3) by the level and consistency of individual and collective feelings about what is wanted and what is tolerable, i.e., the basis of moral suasion or support for any type of implementation, as well as origin, of

Box 7.8. Reasons for VE and MS Failures

- If carried to extremes, **VE** can lead to sizable groups holding to bizarre or violent codes of action that are intolerable to sizable minorities or to the vast majority
- It is probably an obstacle to the use of planning as a flexible vehicle for re-examining problems, selection of new ends, or use of new means, and keeping citizen receptivity open to better approaches
- It is easy to overshoot the mark and preclude early evaluation or redirection
- It may overpower the concern for legitimate counter-views held by sizable minorities in or out of the industry
- It may force one-issue election campaigning further onto elected policy makers
- It can be a waste of resources in massive duplicatory efforts (Roberts Hospital in Oklahoma)
- It can have remote accountability
- There is no evidence that PSROs have had any significant effects on utilization[61] (although PSROs are established by law, they depend on voluntary activities)

FIGURE 7.1
IMPLEMENTATION OF SOCIAL PUROSES:
MARKET (COMPETITION), GOVERNMENT (CONTROL), AND VOLUNTARY EFFORT

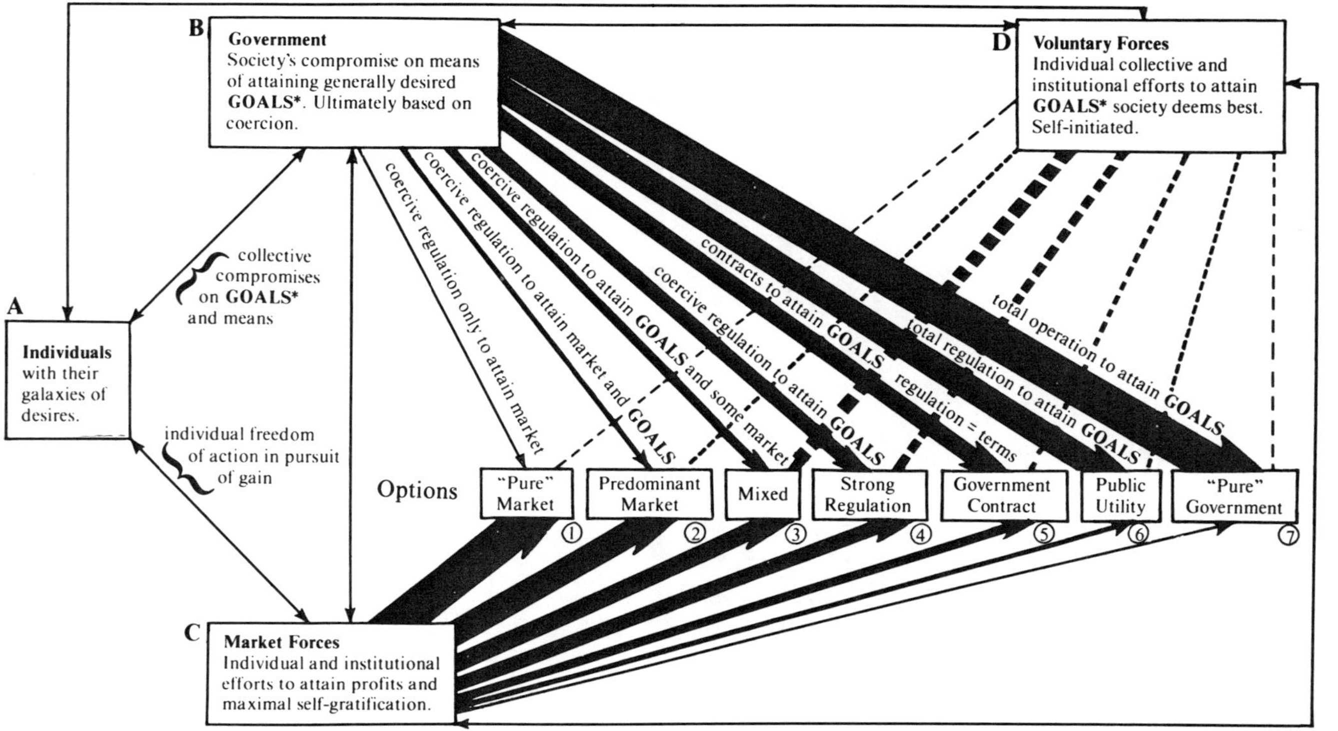

voluntary efforts (**Box D**). The historically-attested inevitability of government, and the frequent erosion or absence of the market, suggest that collectively-based **GOALS** and subsequent regulation are usually predominant, and that market place competition is feared by those in it.

However, the forces of moral suasion either may call for more regulation or for more market-type authority, and for the laws and behavior necessary to attain either. Heavy moral suasion can also lead to voluntary effort and to less dependence on enforcement of any kind, as well as to ease of enforcement. VE may also occur in fields where less than majority groups are free to create something that individuals can't do and governments won't do.

There are seven choices (see **Box 7.9**) that can be made among the policy-implementing options shown on **Figure 7.1.** (Salamon discusses these and others.[62])

It is worth noting that the health sector presently has little, if any, Option 1 settings. It seems that we are currently embarked in moving towards more Option 3 and even some Option 2, and away from heavy dependence on Options 4 or 7, at least for the moment, although County Hospitals (Option 7) are once more being promoted and designated as a source of inexpensive, unpleasant, low-cost care for the poor (AB 799 in California in 1982).

I believe that the discussions so far have made clear the inevitability of providing a layer of government specification (regulations), if we are to achieve any of our purposes, 2) a desirable layer of market-based competition, and 3) a highly-desirable component of voluntary effort. An interesting, eclectic set of cost-containing programs also has emerged from voluntary conjoint efforts of business, labor, providers, and planners, in spite of the present confused and inhospitable legal, and limited market, environment.[63]

B. Inequitable Access to Health Care

This, the second of our major health sector concerns, also has several major causes which we will explore briefly. We will not, however, re-explore the contorted, present-day mix of regulatory, market, and voluntary effort forces which, of course, also underlie the difficulties here.

1. Causes of Inequity

The more immediate causes or intervening variables at work in creating inequities of access are **inappropriate medical specialist training, inadequately-distributed purchasing power, vagaries of coverage for the poor,** and **a combination of rurality, isolation, and lack of amenities.**

Box 7.9. Seven Policy-implementing Options

1. **Pure market** It takes strong, coercive, anti-trust regulation and policing to make sure that there is a market, and that there is no collusion among sellers or among buyers who try to avoid the risks offered by the "pure" competitive market place. In fact, health care seems like a particularly-unsuitable sector to perform reasonably in a heavy market atmosphere, given the **GOALS** it is expected to reach, the history of its development, and consumer-provider relationships over a set or products which is hard to describe or price. The latter factor is one reason that relatively-complete HMO-type services packages, such as "full care for a year" (not unlike a whole automobile), can be priced, and only then can health care services be competitively-marketed for price (see **competition**, pages **165-71**)
2. **Predominatly market (e.g., lots of HMOs)** This differs from the "pure" market in that constraints are placed on the performance of a "pure" market so that **GOALS** will be fairly well delivered. The "pure" market guarantees none of these **GOALS**, not even control of cost, for it may make health care so attractive that the sector grows at an unprecedented rate. As in "pure" market, it takes strong coercive and enabling legislation, and policing, to make sure that there still is a real market. Such **GOAL**-constrained markets work in socialist not-for-profit societies, as well as in profit-oriented capitalistic ones. The pressures, typified by 1982 California laws AB 799, AB 3480 and SB 2012, are setting the stage for active price competition among providers, under a significant layer of regulation
3. **Mixed** This envisions retention of as much strong market place action as compatible with a) strong VE or moral suasion, sponsored by government as well as by producer and buyer elements, and b) use of coercive and enabling regulation to assure avoidance of over-building, guaranteeing quality and safety of products, etc. Coercive regulation exists to guarantee a) lots of market place competition as well as b) introducing specific controls to assure various **GOALS**. The market must be made to produce products wanted, delivery where needed, etc. (not just what and where profitable). It must be understood that regulation may use rewards as well as punishments to achieve its intentions. Regulation is intended to avoid waste by foolish and faddish investments, ensure participation of all consumers so the rest of us don't have to pay their bills when they are sick and broke, etc. There may be heavy reliance on private not-for-profits to overcome the hazards posed by for-profits, as is the case now in our major dependence on non-profit acute care hospitals
4. **Heavy regulation (about where the U.S. was with CON, PSRO, and so on)** This state of affairs means that less is left to market or VE efforts (although PSRO is still mostly VE), and that coercive and enabling legislation and policing determines production and utilization. It could mean strict policing of the market activities that continue (as FTC and anti-trust efforts, which are just now beginning in the health care field)
5. **Government contract (e.g. Medicare and Medicaid).** Use of contracts to preclude "pure" market; allow one large buyer, e.g. government, to write terms which include rewards and punishments, and depends on heavy policing to assure delivery of what is paid for. The only market aspects left are producers fulfilling the contract terms, and making their best efforts to turn a "profit" within the regulating stipulations
6. **Public utility (e.g. American Telephone and Telegraph [AT&T])** Large, otherwise potentially-monopolistic private producers or firms exist under enabling and coercive legislation, which determines their products, quality, safety, competition, distribution, expenditures, costs, prices, income, and profits. This cuts innovation in distribution, does much redistribution of wealth (substitutes somewhat for formal taxation), guarantees **GOALS** to degree desired (some doubts about cost control, profits), and ends most of market competition

   If utilities fail to cooperate or live up to requirements, or go broke, government can take over, restructure, etc. depending on how the enabling legislation is written

Box 7.9. (continued)

7. **Government production (e.g. Veterans Administration [V.A.])** Government itself produces the product, under enabling legislation; its coercive and rewarding regulations are primarily directed at behavior of its own employees, and to "rights of consumers" *vis-a-vis* the service. Government, as a non-profit entity, may produce and "sell" the product in a way that brings in more or less revenue than it costs to operate
   Another form of government production is the quasi-public independent corporation, set up by government to trade, produce, buy, and sell one or many products (such as Tennessee Valley Authority [T.V.A.]); it may be more like for-profit business than it is like government, except that it does not distribute profits directly to owners or stockholders

Unsuitable specialist training The unrealistic medical training patterns of the past 30 years that were spawned by research support and research-oriented faculties turned out too many surgical and super-specialists and too few family-oriented practitioners. This trend is only now being slowed. The non-family-oriented specialists are, for the most part, trained so narrowly that they need a large service area population to support their expertise. They also are trained to be highly dependent on very technologically-advanced equipment and on immediate availability of a full roster of all the specialties. This background precludes their practicing in sparsely-populated areas, and also renders their conversion into generalists most unlikely, even if they do not have enough demands to keep them busy as specialists.[64]

Inadequate purchasing power One of the most aggravating features of our current system of care is the continuing availability of care in accordance with a person's means. In spite of the significantly enlarged financial access provided by Medicare and Medicaid, there still continues to be many millions of our population who get much less care than average, and even less of what they need because of poverty.[65]

The better coverage provided by insurance and Medicare and Medicaid, unfortunately, was not accompanied by any reorganizations of delivery systems of personnel changes in the outputs of medical training centers. This caused significant inflation, which hurt access for the remaining uncovered poor, and led to less coverage for those under Medicare and Medicaid, as well. In addition, the heavy input of new care monies in the late sixties hastened the exodus of urban-ghetto practioners, and did nothing to attract providers to rural areas.[66]

The missing or delayed preventive and therapeutic services for the urban poor, and for many rural persons, whether poor or not, may account for part of their extensive disability and heavy use of hospitalization.

It is of interest that the low utilization of Medicare among the sparsely-populated rural areas has the effect of draining money away from the poorer states to the benefit of the wealthier ones. And Medicaid, thanks to the failure of some poorer states to meet its matching provisions, also drains resources from the poorer rural states to the wealthier urban ones.[67]

The two- and three-fold differences between the physician-population ratios of the better-off states and the poorer ones is a direct reflection of the joint effects of poverty and rurality. The differences in physician-population ratios, of course, are remarkably worse between localities than between states. Many less-well served areas continue to experience a worsening practitioner-population ratio.[68]

Shifting financial eligibility People who move in and out of employment, of course, are at risk of being without coverage much of the time.[69] Going on to Medicaid, as one runs out of private insurance, is not always so simple because of necessary spend-down provisions which may make one almost bankrupt in order to become eligible for Medicaid.

Even worse are the vagaries of Medicaid eligibility, because no two states have the same rules and, often enough, counties doing the eligibility for their state do not enforce the requirements equally. In addition, the Federal and state administrators continue to juggle eligibility each year to cut costs, avoid abuses, and so on, so that all that can be depended on is continued confusion.

The continued and growing gross underpayment of providers further precludes access to many, if not most, providers for those who are fully Medicaid eligible. The geographic unavailability of HMOs also tends to make them inaccessible to most Medicaid eligibles, in the cases where HMOs are allowed to and are willing to take such persons.[70]

It is worth noting that the inequities of access for the poor are no small factor in producing their attendance in Emergency Rooms (where these are available) at a cost of two to four times that for a doctor visit.

Rurality, isolation, and inability to attract practitioners People who live in small towns and rural areas, who are not within easy travel to a major city, are not able to attract doctors. Their old generalists are retiring and dying, and their practitioner-population ratio is dropping. Their population is not large enough to support the customary urban consortium of even basic specialists. Fortunately, as a result of the marked overproduction of specialist physicians, there finally has been a drift of the less-specialized specialists, such as internists, ophthalmologists, general surgeons, and others, to smaller communities of several thousand persons. However, the small communities of one or two thousand persons, or less, are not particularly helped by this scatter of specialists.[71] The hoped-for family physician is just now being trained in reasonable numbers, and in California this has begun to decline once more.[72] However, this modern practitioner, who is appropriately motivated and trained, will not be comfortable working in isolation without some sort of connected system that makes it possible to move patients to specialist care, that makes it possible to take educational leave, and to have recreational relief on a reasonably regular basis.

Rurality, isolation, and lack of connectivity to full health care resources are important obstacles to attracting primary care practitioners. In this connection, it is evident that the northern, fairly-well off, rural tier of states is almost as poorly served as the rural, impoverished, southern ones.[73]

Other threats to the underserved, such as the malpractice insurance mess Currently, the malpractice burden is falling heavily on the older and less-active physicians and on the family practitioners who do a wide variety of services and pay premiums relevant to the most-costly insurance element of their practice, such as obstetrics. The poor and the isolated areas are just the ones that have more than their share of such physicians, and many of these are now giving up practice because of insurance costs. Physicians that have many Medicaid patients, in particular, are being driven out of practice since they are increasingly-poorly renumerated and cannot afford an additional five to twenty thousand dollar annual insurance penalty. Young practitioners cannot go into such practices because such sizable insurance costs represent serious additional obstacles to normally significant start-up costs.

As an offset, the availability of physicians for work in city and county health services is going up as a consequence of the complexities of private practice. The same is true for the National Health Service Corps. But these represent miniscule additions, many of which are poorly financed and organized, and often only modestly productive compared to the physicians in private practice.

2. The Possibilities for Improvement of Access

The HCDS The utilization of organized HCDSs to bracket the nation, as part of a nationally-funded health care scheme, will take care of two major obstacles. HCDSs can attract physicians and other health care providers (of which there is a growing glut) by means of favorable work, living, and insurance arrangements.[74] They offer an ideal means of financing care for the disadvantaged and well-off alike. They also create the incentives for cost and quality control through prospectively-negotiated per-capita financing, as from a National Health Pool for all the health services care of a designated group of subscribers.

Primary Care Providers The continued improvements in selection and in primary care education will help reach our underserved, particularly when combined with the necessary financing and organization of delivery.[75]

C. Our Unacceptable Health Status

The most damning thing that can be said about the world's best-endowed and richest country is that not only is it not the leader in health status, but that recently it only has been holding its own in the ranks of the major nations. In 1979, the U.S. ranked **7th** among the top 16 industrialized capitalist nations of the world in life expectancy at birth, and **12th** in infant mortality.[76] This needs explaining before we can rectify it. More importantly, huge variations in health status are evident in the U.S. from one place to the next, and from one group to the next.[77]

1. Explanation of our unequal health status at home and our poor showing among the nations of the world.

What is certain is that only two or three other countries spend as much as we do per capita for medical, i.e., sickness care. What also is certain is that the care available is technically among the best, even if used too lavishly, and thus dangerously. However, it is also quite clear that none of the countries which stand above us in health status have such a high proportion of medically-disenfranchised persons as we do. Given the evidence already presented, that medical care is not that valuable and that the access to it is not that bad, it seems most unlikely that the significant proportion of our population who get few health services is the only cause of our bad health status showing.

Several other hypotheses have more explanatory power. These fall into two categories: 1) **excessive poverty,** both actual and relative, and 2) **excessive affluence** (see **Chapters 1-3,** regarding inputs to health).

Excessive poverty, actual and relative These conditions probably are more prevalent in the U.S. than in any of the countries that have a better infant mortality rate and female life expectancy at birth. This probably is true also for all but four or five of the countries with a longer life expectancy in males. In the notably-poor countries that do very well healthwise, some of which exceed us in male survival, difficult living conditions are a more-accepted way of life. A good basic diet, basic medical care, basic education, and life-long employment opportunities are an everyday fact of life. In the U.S., a national unemployment level of ten percent is likely to be 30 percent in the ghetto, while the rest of the community is usually less than five percent. The unforgettable, everyday reminders of ethnic handicaps, such as school riots, particularly affect the same disadvantaged peoples as do crime, drug abuse, and school dropouts. All of these probably result from, and compound, the mixture known as deprivation. The countries that have surpassed us in health do not have such severe or entrenched socio-economic problems. Nor are such a high proportion of their people involved in them.

Excessive affluence This factor may not seem so obvious as a cause of ill-health. But a little reflection and review of data on life expectancy trends of adults suggest that it is probably another cause for our poor showing (see **Chapter 3**). Colloquially speaking, few other nations can afford such unhealthful ways of living. Each of our affluence-propelled, anti-health, behavioral deficits somehow presents itself as an attractive life style. Excessive intake of animal protein and fats, dangerous imbibing habits of alcohol, tobacco, and drugs (prescribed and proscribed), dangerous recreational sports and driving habits, are all possible because of affluence.

Moreover, our heritage, desires, opportunities, and our "macho," combined with the relatively low cost and omnipresent availability and attractiveness of bad foods and speedy vehicles, makes us particularly vulnerable to our affluence. And those in our society who aren't affluent "try harder."

2. Means for Improvement of Health Status

The possibilities for improvement fall into several different categories. Each, as it will be seen, is more easily approached if all persons are cared for in a PWC, which is part of an HCDS (see **Figure 4.3**, page **89**).

Specific anti-failure measures Several measures come to mind from what has been offered in the way of explanations of ill-health. A direct attack is needed on the specific elements that go into creating the adverse health status of those communities or groups which today fall below the national average. For example, just raising them to the average for infant death rate (which is still inferior to what other neighboring communities now achieve) would put us in the forefront of the nations for life expectancy at birth. Examples of success are provided in both developing and in developed countries. Enormous improvements have been effected by the use of not overly-elaborately trained workers (students, nurses etc.), providing pregnant women or hypertensives with outreach, caring, advice, support, or advocacy, with a modicum of medical supervision.[78]

Combination of somatic, psychic, and social primary services Based on ecologic perceptions of what is involved in maintaining and restoring health, it has become imperative that persons who "hurt," for whatever reason, have reasonable access to a source of support to those practitioners who have comprehension and incentives to utilize the approaches that are best calculated to succeed with a given client.

All new primary care developments in the underserved areas must combine the somatic, psychic, and social support services. Typically, all three services are deficient in the same areas, and it is in just the underserved areas where the greatest and the most uncared-for somatic, psychic, and social needs exist in their most mutually-aggravating forms.

Fundamental macro-ecologic measures (need for equalization of opportunities for the disadvantaged) Reorganization and reconceptualization of health care is still far from being the most significant approach to a rapid equalization of our eminently unequal health status. Once and for all, we will have to deliver the same opportunity structure and environment for the bottom quarter as we do for middle America. One of the simplest ways of doing this would be by rebuilding our central city ghettoes, and by providing each family with the opportunity for ownership of the unit they live in so as to give them a stake in it. Irrespective of whether they are on relief or not, they can buy subsidized housing just as easily as they can rent it. The importance of this approach to good health also carries the promise of an effective attack on urban disintegration, with its abuse, neglect, degeneracy, homicide, suicide, crime, blighted childhood, drugged and boozed teens, and alienated adults.

Another approach worth exploring is to "buy out" adverse, but heretofore legitimate interests, such as those which pollute us through our water, air, soil, or food. We could begin a non-adversary approach to such matters, i.e. buying out a taconite lake polluter, or buying out the tobacco or alcohol advertising business. "Buying out" includes planning and financing new uses for plants and workers in hazard-producing industries, so that a victory for one group's health is not replaced by disaster for another's.

Primary health care can also add many things of value which it does not now commonly offer Having already presented the rationale in **Chapters 1-6,** we can briefly list what good, close-at-hand, primary care could be structured to do that would add to well-being. The list includes:

1. an advocacy posture in behalf of a given client with problems of any consequence
2. a connectivity function in relation to all the client's needed support services
3. a sharing or partnership relationship of a key provider to those clients desiring it
4. a push towards increased client self-determination and self-care
5. a push towards prospective medicine, which evaluates the

clients' strengths and weaknesses and helps them towards healthier behaviors specifically relevant to them

6. encouragement for client participation in governance of prepaid health care delivery systems and in health planning efforts
7. helping clients into a macro-ecologic and health-relevant, world-political outlook, so that their combined interests help set the stage for an environment that is more and more fit to live in[79]
8. helping subscribers attain a personal or micro-ecologic perspective which incorporates respect for their own needs, and for the generally hazardous behaviors and environments over which they can exert some control

Tying the physicians' welfare to that of their clients and subscribers The physicians' economic welfare must be tied to that of their patients, so that they care:

1. that their patients' physical living, work, and recreation environments do not cause them needless illness
2. that their patients' socio-educational environment does not encourage behavioral traps, such as extensive use of alcohol and tobacco
3. that their patients are educated and encouraged to make use of the well-tried preventive procedures, the use of which is kept free of any obvious barriers
4. that patients are encouraged to check out their own vulnerabilities and be guided to healthy behavior, accordingly
5. that there are suitable levels of care in facilities and at home, so that no sick person need be sent to needlessly-sophisticated and expensive facilities
6. that all persons have access to any of the care systems in their area, and have free choice among them
7. that there is an adequate variety of care systems, so people can get into the ones they best fit[80]
8. that anti-disease endeavors are explored that may involve services at places of employment, stores, or schools.[81]

This can only be expected to take place when pre-negotiated, annually-fixed sums of money are provided to complete health systems for the totality of health services for a given group of subscribers who participate in a PWC providing psychic, somatic, and social services, and who share in the governance of their system. There the incentives for thrift are built in, because intervening in the right places at the right time by the right kind of intervener is to everyone's advantage.[82] And what is saved can be shared among the providers as well as subscribers.

It is in this setting that the several diverse meanings of quality can be brought together, and all achieved. Covell describes two related concepts: 1) acceptable level of practices in a community, and 2) the degree of excellence attainable, relative to the state of the art.[83] Both of these focus on technical adequacy, but neither even hint at two other critical areas: 1) what the care does for health status, and 2) what the level of caring is.[84]

III. A NATIONAL POLICY PROPOSAL FOR HEALTH AND HEALTH CARE

A. The Five Goals: Recapitulation

The major health sector problems of increasing cost, inequitable access, and inadequate health status call for five major goals if we are to take advantage of what we know and what we have at the lowest feasible cost in money, energy, and political disharmony, and emerge with a satisfactory health and health care situation. The five major goals are:

1. **Wisely use what we already have**
2. **Achieve cost control of health care, and thereby provide adequate resources for improving health and equitable access**
3. **Achieve equity in distribution of health care**
4. **Achieve improvement of health status**
5. **Reformulate health care by adding new health-promoting roles to the health care system**

B. What is Needed: the Methods Required to Reach the Five Goals, the Standards at Which to Aim, (and by Which to Gauge Our Accomplishments), and Implementation

It would be handy if each of the five goals could be amplified into specific sub-objectives, each of which could then be assigned appropriate methodologies. However, we can only proceed safely if we lay out the system, or abstract model of health care, taking care to subdivide it as realistically as possible and to delineate its practical boundaries. Then we can suggest how to affect each part of the system needing it, so that, as a totality, it moves satisfactorily towards our stipulated five goals. **Figure 7.2** is a model of the overall health care delivery system, which allows us to point out what needs to be done in each major part of the delivery system, and between the various parts of the national health care endeavor.

1. Organization: the creation and provision of services

Health dollars provided for services do not, by themselves, create the best or wisest use, organization, or direction of the delivery services. We anticipate creating more expensive, and worse, failures in equity and health, if the dollars go out indiscriminately to bolster existing service mechanisms. The "National Moratorium" on facilities and services, to be discussed under financing, is a key step to reaching our goals.

FIGURE 7.2
A WORKING MODEL FOR THE HEALTH CARE DELIVERY SYSTEM (HCDS)

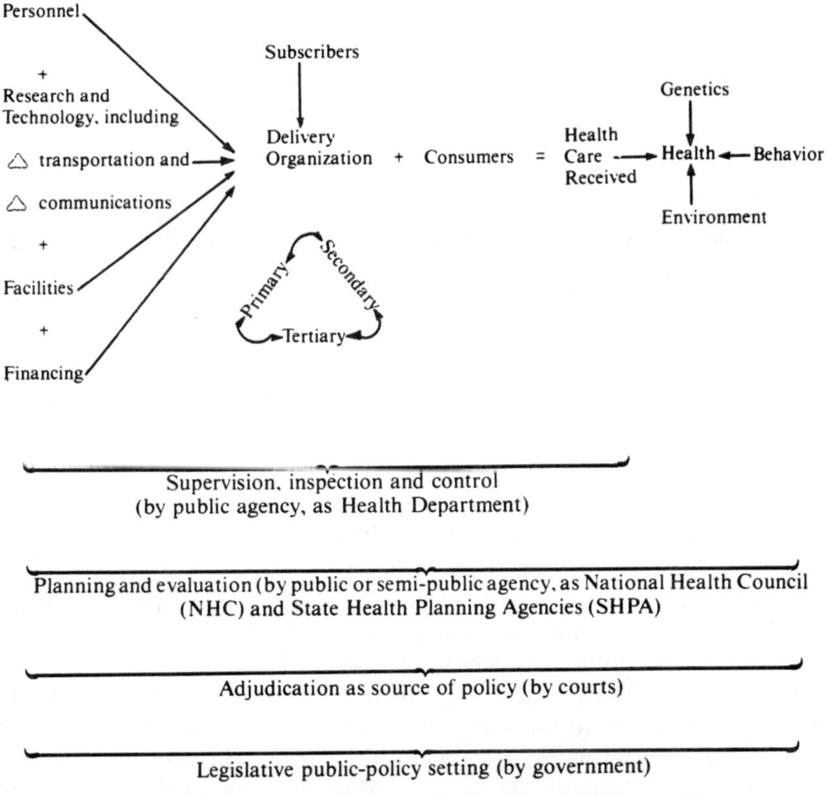

Adapted from H. L. Blum, *Planning for Health*, Human Sciences Press, 2nd Edition, 1981, p. 183.

Every person will have a well-defined package of prepaid care available from an organized Health Care Delivery Systems (HCDS) In 1983-84, each State Health Planning Agency (SHPA) entity, or its local subdivision, would determine the extent to which each HCDS would provide coverage, and what it would have to do in the way of providing services to the adjacent underserved areas so that everyone in the state would have at least one conveniently-accessible and acceptable HCDS.

A comprehensive, fully-prepaid package of services will be made available to every person residing in the U.S. in 1984-85, through a reasonably-accessible HCDS as approved by the SHPA. There will be only modest, income-graduated and prevention-excepted co-payments, and thus the earliest, as well as the most-prolonged, catastrophic care will be covered.

HCDSs must be built up from small primary care delivery units or well-being centers (PWCs) located near to consumers. Their services are based on primary care provided through their PWCs, serving from 2,000 to 10,000 persons each, and must be as significantly diverse as consumer choice and utilization requires.[85] HCDSs probably cannot function well with less than 30,000 subscribers, and should generally serve 50,000 or more. Multiple, modest-sized HCDSs in any given area are preferable to large monopolistic ones. The SHPA will guide size, distribution, and diversity.

A comprehensive package of connected somatic and psychic services Every HCDS must offer a complete package of services as broad as called for in the original Health Maintenance Organization law (HMO PL 93-222). By 1986, each HCDS must include all long-term somatic, psychic, and mental retardation services as are needed. In extenuating circumstances, as approved by the SHPA, the package could be built up over a period to 1988.

Combined somatic, psychic, and social primary services in all underserved areas where new services and facilities have to be created Initially, creation of entirely new services and facilities will be allowed only for the underserved areas or groups, as specified by the SHPA. In the underserved areas requiring any new facilities or services, all somatic, psychic, and social services will be combined at each of the PWCs. The combination or pooling of all the human support dollars in one pre-negotiated pot, for all the subscribers, will provide the incentives for the served community, with assistance of the various providers involved, to work out cost-effective ways of organizing one-stop, promotive, preventive, diagnostic, therapeutic, and rehabilitative services for individuals and families.

The SHPA will undertake the necessary brokerage and planning for the combined human services in underserved areas, and indicate when it approves of the combined services proposal, which will justify the expenditures from the national pool for any new services and facilities.

Quality controls These will not be adequately successful if based on peer review focused on structure and process. Such procedures fail not only to take into account patient and institution participation in the care process, but have great difficulty in including scrutiny of outpatient or office care. The scrutiny of outcomes in a statistical way, and analysis of each bad outcome for causative factors, is more valuable and probably much-less costly in the long run.[86] This scrutiny should be done by the SHPA or its local arm, if there is one. It is also our belief that effective cost control under pre-negotiated per-capitation will spill over into better choices about care, and into considerations of outcome. Cost controlling will be a positive incentive and have good effects on our quest for a continuing improvement in quality. Quality will take on dimensions of health, and health care will be scrutinized for what it does for health. The various approaches now under study for use in quality control and possibilities of technology assessment would be continued at the present 1982 level of PSRO expenditures, and must be treated purely as experimentation, not to be extended until better methods are documented.[87] Incompetency or dishonesty in practice will be ferreted out by the quality machinery. Consumer-dominated boards of both the PWCs and HCDSs will make determinations about professional suitability and caring in their settings. Malpractice issues will be resolved by new forms of more widely-based insurance against injury and against loss of function or income, or at least by inclusion in the overall medical care financing.

2. Subscriber and consumer participation.

There are three major concerns here:

Subscriber participation in policy and governance Subscribers make up the element of the health care system which is usually taken for granted. They need an immediate and direct voice in decisions about purposes, shaping modes of service, coverage, finance, terms of remuneration, and facilities.[88] When subscribers become consumers, they also need to be actively involved in their own care decisions to the extent they wish. Subscriber involvement in HCDS governance must be restructured to include a preponderance of representatives from organized, and particularly from disadvantaged, heavy-user, consumer groups, such as aged, disabled, parents, gays, women, poor, Native Americans, Blacks, Chicanos, and so on.

Subscriber participation in macro- and micro-ecologic orientations If subscribers are to "consume" what is most valuable to them, in terms of societal policy decisions and personal behavior decisions, they must become more active participants in what the HCDSs have to offer in the way of macro- and micro-ecologic orientations, and how the two interrelate.[89] This includes subscriber opportunity to participate in studies regarding their community and their personal health,[90] participation in planning and design of educational programs, and so on.

Consumer participation in care Consumers of care must have a major role in participating in the care process, because they can do or undo much of the care they ask for and receive. They have to learn how to be a partner with their practitioner, make decisions they can and will live with, do as much of their own care as is reasonable, accept care from family and friendly neighbors who will help them use and carry out appropriate services prescribed by the practitioner, and, in turn, assist in the care of others. They need to, and happily can, learn how to be more self-sufficient, and release practitioners to do the tasks for which they (practitioners) are most needed.

3. Financing: the collection and distribution of dollars for services

Some six major areas must be taken into account here:

A national cost ceiling, and specified health improvement fund which, in 1983-84, totals 12 percent of the GNP of the prior year The first step is to declare our objective of holding the overall annual health sector costs each year to no more than a fixed proportion of the GNP. For the year 1983-84, I would suggest that it be ten percent of the GNP of the preceding year, 1982-83. The health care costs *per se*, including construction, must be held to no more than nine percent of GNP, so that the one percent of GNP for public health programs, health personnel education, and research would not be squeezed out by medical care.

An additional two percent of GNP will be set aside each year to invest in health-improving measures, as prioritized by the National Health Council (NHC), which has more significant duties than the one set up by P. L. 93-641. This brings the entire health sector budget to 12 percent of GNP. If we do not set a finite ceiling and stick to it, we will experience a continued escalation of the percent of GNP going primarily for sickness care. When we wrote the first edition of this book, only six years ago, we were able to say that eight percent of GNP should go to care and two percent to create health. Of course, our nation never set an eight percent lid on care, and it never allocated two percent of the GNP for new monies to build a healthier, happier, and more prosperous country. Now, just a few years later, we are at ten percent for care, which has absorbed the once proposed two percent for creating health.

When will we call a halt to increasing sickness care, and start using that extra bit of resources to create health (less sickness)? The two percent for health would give us more employment by creating better housing, lower energy and safer transport, schools, recreation, and clean cities, all routes to better health and a more-fun existence. Yes, moving such monies to the sickness arena also gives us jobs, but they attend only casualties and build but little for health.

A national health care services dollar-pool Beginning in 1983-84, all health dollars are collected into one national pool. The dollars initially are derived 25 percent from general revenues to guarantee some progressive redistribution, and 75 percent from employment (social-security type) taxes on the first $35,000 of income to guarantee funding stability. Those with an income not under social security, and the self-employed, would also match the employment tax as well by paying income tax. Each year, after 1984-85, the percent derived from general revenues would shift up five percent, and from social security down five percent, until stabilized at 50 percent each in 1990.

The monies in the care services pool are distributed to each HCDS according to the number of subscribers, taking into account age and poverty as well as local variations in costs of services. These are global budgets, essentially block grants, except that in contrast to those of the Reagan Administration, they will contain the needed monies for complete health services for each HCDS and for every person in the U.S.

All other health care funding mechanisms are absorbed Medicare and Medicaid, as well as all other special categories of eligibles for whatever reason, such as Indians, Federal employees, or veterans, would be shifted into the national pool in 1984-85. In 1985-86, the states, cities, and counties would be eliminated from any participation in the costs of acute care, and, by 1986-87, from all institutional care for physical, mental, or emotional conditions.

Agencies of government would be eligible to maintain an HCDS, or a service operation meeting the nation's HCDS standards, and would receive from the national pool the same pre-negotiated, per-capita payments for the care they provide. They could also become partners or contractors in services provided by any HCDS.

Start-up costs made available Encouragement in the form of an initial 90 percent subsidy from the national pool, for construction and purchase of facilities and equipment would be available to systems serving underserved areas, when so certified by the SHPA. In areas certified by the

SHPA as poverty areas which are without adequate facilities in accordance with NHC national standards, 100 percent of the facility costs would be met. Unused former government facilities, where appropriate, would be assigned by SHPA.

When approved by the SHPA, the initial organizing costs of an HCDS and the costs of starting new services would be met from the national pool on the basis of formulae worked out by the National Health Council (NHC).

The advantages of Independent Practice Association (IPA) models, utilizing existing practitioners and facilities, over setting up new groups with new facilities, need to be emphasized. Insignificant start-up costs, freedom of choice for subscriber, and maximal freedom for the practitioner, are all advantages of this model over the closed-panel groups.

A national moratorium on capital outlay and new services, to enable catching-up in the underserved areas In order to assure adequate catch-up of the have-not areas, new facilities or equipment not already on order or under construction, are not allowed anywhere in the U.S. until all the underserved areas, as certified by the SHPA (according to the 1983 NHC definitions of underserved) are brought up to acceptable local coverage for primary care and the ability to offer the complete care package. New services and facilities are allowed in any area where the full package otherwise could not be offered, and where an HCDS reaches into an underserved area that requires additional services and facilities. Replacement of defective equipment and basic facility and equipment maintenance would continue.

New services and facilities after the moratorium Once the SHPA certified that all underserved groups were brought up to suitable service levels like everyone else, new activities would be permitted in accordance with SHPA plans. The costs of SHPA-permitted expansions and replacements would be included in the pre-negotiation for the per-capita reimbursement to each HCDS. However, for other than research purposes, nothing would be permitted or erected that was not SHPA-approved, no matter what the source of funding.

4. Personnel

Health personnel is probably the most critical element in providing services, but, unfortunately, as experience has taught us, it does not stand alone.[91] The government's role in this area generally has run counter to controlling costs or providing the needed manpower. It has to be integrated into the national policy.

Training and subsidization National support to professional schools for training health professionals essentially has been phased out by 1982. But national pool resources would be set aside to fund training for those categories of health professionals, such as primary care physicians and mid-level practitioners, which SHPA and NHC studies point out are going to be in short supply for ten or more years unless given special support. Because some regions have different shortages than others, specific regional policies for subsidization may have to be made by the NHC. The ultimate pattern of financing all health-provider training will be worked out by the National Health Council.

National pool support for individuals receiving training in subsidized programs would be available for tuition and living expenses. Anyone accepting such support will have no choice but to put in a period of service for each year of professional training at the national average income for that profession in an "open," i.e. under-manned, area. There will be no way to cancel this obligation (see **Licensure,** below).

Designated quotas for advanced training in medicine The NHC, working with the AMA, AHA, and the medical specialty boards, will develop for each specialty a quota of training opportunities by 1984. These will be distributed suitably over the country and be updated every two years as indicated.

Licensure *Temporary* licensure for physicians (MD) and osteopaths (DO) will be nationwide for new graduates and, initially, will be based on passage of National Boards for MDs. National Boards will be extended to other providers in the same way. *Permanent* licensure will be granted to individuals in accordance with evidence that they have provided designated services called for by their acceptance of educational support. Providers already in practice will be granted national licenses if their state licensure meets national standards.

The National Health Council will set up a study commission to review National Board licensure examinations to be constructed around performance testing. The commission will also investigate the utility of periodic re-examinations. It will work out a means of licensing HCDSs so that on the basis of performance and outcome measures they may utilize personnel innovatively in any way that meets such standards, irrespective of professional licensure restrictions. All these changes should be in effect by 1986-87.

Recruitment and equity Equity between sexes and ethnics in career opportunities is not only a moral obligation in a democracy, but is becoming more and more a necessity if services are to be acceptable to women and minorities. Recruitment of potentially-suitable candidates for the professions, who are likely to work where needed and whose training is to be subsidized, should become a responsibility of SHPAs or their local arms.[92] Acceptance of recruits by professional schools would be a joint responsibility of the SHPA and the schools receiving related subsidies. This principle should be extended to all health career lines by 1986-87.

5. Facilities and equipment

This area calls for two sets of constraints which work in somewhat opposed ways, if sensible solutions are to be achieved.

Restraint The ludicrous super-abundance of the acute secondary and tertiary facilities in many parts of the U.S. has to be "grown into." Part of it can be utilized for primary care purposes where needed, some for extended care, and some of it as institutional low-cost rest homes or hotels for the enfeebled. The moratorium already described will enable the planners and architects to review the demands that organized care systems make on SHPAs, so that when the moratorium is over and new facilities are requested they can be more relevantly located, designed, and constructed.

Redundancy is not wholly evil Just as a super-abundance is a waste of our resources, so an over-zealous approach to efficiency, and insistence on heavy usage of any given facility or equipment, may harm the usefulness, choice, acceptability, and even the efficiency of the whole system. Similarly, insistence on fewer very large, rather than on more smaller facilities, may inhibit innovation and even introduce serious inefficiencies, as well as private costs, to consumers.

6. Research and technologic advances

Support from the national pool would be available at a level determined by the National Health Council, through the National Science Foundation and the National Institutes of Health, on a modified peer review basis. Other contributed funds could be used in any way desired by researchers, within the usual criteria laid down by institutional and ethical constraints.

It is suggested that first priority go to "decisive" technology, as described by Thomas.[93] The second priority should go to "simple" technology for extending self-help, and for use by unsophisticated health workers. The third priority should go to "mid-level" technology, which currently gets the lion's share of research funds and is utilized to reconstruct victims after disaster strikes; and therefore occasions the most-costly and least-productive health care. It is worth quoting Mechanic, who says, *In the final analysis, the success of medical care must be measured by what is achieved in the aggregate rather than in its scientific elegance or its more miraculous achievements.*[94]

There should be continued NHC review of the research policy affecting health, as for all the other policy matters. The proposed division between research, education, and services, as well as the allocations between the research levels, as proposed here, would be revised annually.

7. Roles of health departments

As the state and local government provision of somatic and psychic services will be turned over to HCDSs, with financing provided from the national pool. The roles of health departments will have been altered drastically by these changes.

Surveillance over health care It would seem wise to maintain health departments in an operations surveillance role over HCDSs to assure the scope and quality of their performance. Whether local health departments should participate in this role, or whether it should be restricted to state health departments is a decision that deserves studying, and one that may vary from state to state. In any case, surveillance should not become the function of any of the levels (national, state, or regional) of planning bodies.

Environmental surveillance and control Overseeing the quality of various aspects of the environment is an already badly-fractionated and dispersed set of services at every level of government, and varies from place to place. No prescription can be made at this time as to the role of health departments in this area.

The National Health Council will replan the roles of health departments In the 1985 86 National Health Policy to be submitted by the NHC, a proposal should be made for the distribution and financing of the tasks described above under surveillance of care and environment.

8. The roles of the national, state, and sub-state level planning bodies

The NHC and the state (and regional) planning bodies (SHPAs), which were established under PL 93-641, have many broad and many very well-specified tasks. It is our belief that if they survive they need drastic modification.

The NHC drafts the national health policy Beginning in 1984-85, and every year thereafter, the NHC will plan and present an updated national health policy directly to the President for transmission to the Congress and the nation.

The NHC reports directly to the President The importance of the national health policy, and the planning which goes into it, requires that the NHC report directly to the President, and that nominations to it be approved by a Congressionally-designated committee composed of members of both houses. The NHC cannot be the handmaiden of the U.S. Department of Health and Human Services (HHS) if it is to have impact or get the staffing needed to do one of the Nation's more important tasks.

The NHC prepares the national health pool budget The NHC already has the task of helping design the national health policy, for which this policy proposal was meant to offer suggestions. The NHC should be given the further task of converting the National Health Policy into a budget proposal.

The NHC convenes the SHPAs annually, prior to presenting its policy and budget recommendations Before the NHC presents its annual policy and budget update to Congress and to the President, it needs to hold a two-week workshop with representatives from each SHPA. This would provide the opportunity for an airing not otherwise likely to take place, particularly of the bottom-up recommendations which the SHPAs need to make to the NHC about various state needs and priorities.

The NHC analyzes the nation's major health problems and designs workable approaches With its own staffing, and with further assistance from HHS, the NHC will undertake the analysis of each of the major causes of premature death and disability for each age group. This will be done in terms of the forces at work: 1) the macro-ecologic environmental forces that are far beyond the control of individuals or their health care, 2) the micro-ecologic environmental and behavioral forces which can be influenced by an individual or family and their source of health care, 3) genetic contributions, and 4) health care contributions, *per se*, which are or could be routinely available in every HCDS.

The NHC is expected to develop appropriate mixes or packages of interventions against our major health threats, based on their comparative effectivity, feasibility, cost, acceptability, and so on. The NHC is required to utilize all of its influence in making the nation aware of its recommendations, and is given 0.1 percent of the national health pool with which to do so.

The NHC will undoubtedly have the most difficulty in finding the necessary support for the macro-ecologic interventions which have the most to do with health, such as occupational safety, clean air, clean water, full employment, low energy transport, city rebuilding, and so on. However, the two percent of the GNP which is to be spent on programs created under NHC leadership to accomplish this purpose will provide some remarkable incentives.

The NHC reviews all major national legislative and program proposals for "health impact" As a start towards intersectoral coordination, all major national legislative and programmatic proposals, and particularly those involving the U.S. Departments of Housing and Urban Development (HUD), Health and Human Services (HHS), Transportation (DOT), the Environmental Protection Agency (EPA), and the Energy Resource Development Agency (ERDA), must be reviewed by the NHC. Although exerting no decision-making power in this area, the NHC will advise the President and the Congress on probable "health impacts" of proposed legislation over the short and long run.[95]

The NHC reviews and approves the work plan and budget for the national collection of health and service data to be used in planning The NHC reviews and approves the linked efforts of such bodies as the Cooperative Health Statistics System and the office of Research and Statistics. It will oversee development of health indices, measurement approaches, data collection and analysis procedures, and the creation of a nationwide health data base for the nation's planning activities.[96]

SHPAs are given support for improving health status Using NHC guidance. SHPAs will study infant death and age-specific death for the ten major causes of death in their jurisdiction, by socio-economic characteristics and by HCDS membership.

With NHC guidance, each SHPA also will collate evidence on such conditions as alcoholism, smoking, drug abuse, accidents, occupationally-caused conditions, levels of immunization, home safety checks, well-child supervision, use of Pap smears, and gather information about health behavior and environment from data that it specifies be provided by HCDSs and other agencies. It will analyze the data relevant to HCDS practices, socio-economic status, and so on, to develop approaches to intercept or counteract anti-health influences in its jurisdiction. Each SHPA will have an amount equal to one percent of the dollars for health care in its state to award to HCDSs or other community agencies for activities it determines are suitable for introducing needed changes, consumer incentives, and so on. The efforts so funded will be reveiwed annually and renegotiated annually. Each SHPA will have another similar amount to utilize in initiating health-promoting activities.

The proposals just presented resemble in many ways the ongoing scheme in Canada, where roughly half of all health service funds are Federally-generated and then redistributed to the provinces along population, age, and wealth guidelines. The provinces act somewhat like HMOs (HCDS), making sure that all aspects of care are available for all of their citizens. For the most part, provinces utilize prospectively-negotiated, fee-for-service rates with practitioner organizations, and prospective budgeting with individual facilities. Canada also is one of the few countries with essentially total coverage, essentially no co-payments, broad mental health coverage, and a health sector bill well below that in the U.S.; above all, one which continues to take a declining share of the Canadian GNP.[97] Others have come up with analyses and schemes that share some features in common with those presented here.[98]

IV. REALISTICALLY, WHAT CAN WE EXPECT TO GET IN THE WAY OF EFFECTIVE POLICY?

Whatever one may think of the American credo, one perceives that it leads politicans to offer promises which are only haltingly and partially matched by policy or subsequent legislation. That which does get legislated is seldom organized or funded in a way that could effectively carry out the stated intent. No real changes could have been intended to stem from P. L. 89-749, our first overall health planning venture. P. L.93-641, its successor, offered planning body organization and much process, but little that was calculated to investigate the nature of problems or to instigate change. Its planning bodies were discretely disconnected from affecting the mainstreams of financing or institutional organization which might offer hopes of effecting cost control. They had even less with which to affect the inequities in receipt of care. Their general mandate was at its most oblique when it came to scrutinizing the major socio-economic and physical environmental variables which lie outside the health sector, but which have more effects on health status than anything the health sector can be expected to do by itself.

What are the chances that a meaningful national health policy proposal could get produced and be turned into effective legislation? In spite of how much we would like to control health care costs, satisfy equity in care distribution, and vastly improve our health status, we have a mighty plurality of competing interests and many of the more powerful ones stand to have at least short-run losses from our proposals.[99] Until we work our way out of the special interest approach to achieving legislation, we will probably squirm through many a hopeful and hopeless panacea that avoid real change before we will settle for a coherent and meaningful policy.[100]

Under these circumstances, are there pieces of this policy proposal acceptable enough so that they can be put in line with what we already have, and lead us towards our five goals? We believe there are and we will outline them briefly, after a short preface on financing.

We are convinced of the need for full national financing (collection and distribution) for health services, as part of an extensive reorganization of health services. At the same time, we are opposed to beginning the reorganization effort by the one step of open-ended assumption of health service funding by the Federal government. We feel that taking only the single step of financing would totally undermine our efforts at controlling costs, and thereby fail to create equity of service distribution or improvement of health status. Since we also do not expect any well-thought out effective reorganization of our health services to take place through a single act of political implementation, we would proceed with the policy elements as shown below.

1. Declare a national moratorium on all new capital outlay and services, except where they are absent and needed to make up approved HCDSs (HMOs), or replace worn out equipment. The moratorium would continue until all areas or groups classified by SHPAs as underserved in 1983-84 are fully served by one or more qualified HCDSs, as verified by the SHPA.
2. Encourage the formation of fully-prepaid HCDSs (under the HMO law service standards), with the addition of the organizational and service start-up support suggested in this proposal.
3. Require subscriber participation in the governance of HCDSs, as described earlier.
4. Merge all somatic, psychic, and social primary care services wherever an HCDS is serving an area designated as underserved by the SHPA. The HCDS would receive all the social, psychic, and somatic care funds involved.
5. As soon as the full National Health Policy is in effect, allocate two percent of the GNP annually to attack those major social problems which affect health, as designated by the NHC. While this policy is being developed, establish a pattern of ongoing national debate on resource utilization and health policies.
6. Assign the NHC the task of working out, and getting implementation inside HHS, of a nationwide system of health and service indices, measurements, and data collection.
7. Assign the NHC the task of a) analyzing the ten major causes of death and the ten major causes of disability for the seven major age groupings in terms of the four forces affecting health, and b) of working out the most feasible basic interventions which are to be put in the form of sub-objectives of the National Health Policy. This is to be updated every two years.
8. Provide the SHPAs with an amount equal to one percent of the health care costs in their jurisdiction to undertake health promotion, and another one percent to initiate delivery system changes.
9. Adopt the personnel policies of this proposal.
10. Adopt the research funding policies of this proposal.

11. Provide for Federal take-over of all health care funding functions now carried by local and state governments.

12. Provide for the Federal collection of all health care funds, and redistribution to HCDSs which provide all health care for their subscribers on an annual, pre-negotiated, demographically-adjusted, per-capita basis. Each person in the U.S. annually will select an HCDS of his or her choice which will receive that person's share of care funds. The total of all health service funds will not exceed a stipulated fixed amount, e.g. ten percent, of the GNP of the prior year, and the health care financing portion will not exceed nine percent of the GNP of the prior year. There is simultaneous federal collection of additional health-promoting funds, to the extent of two percent of the GNP of the prior year, which is to be distributed in accordance with NHC plans for promoting health.

REFERENCES

1. *Health Care Issues in the Decade of Scarcity,* Proceedings of the Third Triennial Foster G. McGaw Health Care Conference, Loyola Medical Center, Maywood, Illinois, April 7, 1981. .L. R. Brown, *Building a Sustainable Society,* New York, W. W. Norton, 1981. *World Watch Paper Series,* World Watch Institute, 1776 Massachusetts Avenue, N. W., Washington, D. C., 20036.

2. N. Milio, *Promoting Health Through Public Policy,* Philadelphia, F. D. Davis, 1980.

3. *Medical Care Expenditures, Prices and Costs: Background Book,* Office of Research and Statistics, Washington, D. C., September 1975, DHEW Publication (SSA) 75-11909. *Towards aComprehensive Health Policy for the 1970's,* US DHEW, May 1971, 10-21. J. C. Morreale, "Is National Health Insurance the Best We Can Do?", *Health Policy Quarterly,* Summer 1981, 1:22, 125-141. R. M. Gibson and D. R. Waldo, "National Health Expenditures, 1981," *Health Care Financing Review,* September, 1982, 4:1, 1-36.

4. M. Mesarovic and E. Pestel, *Mankind at the Turning Point,* New York, E. P. Dutton and Co., Inc., 1974. Trend Analysis Program No. 12, Institute of Life Insurance, 277 Park Avenue, New York, Fall 1975. "The Coming Food Crunch," *Cry California,* Summer 1981, 16:4, 6-18. L. Brown, ibid No. 1.

5. "Public Unwilling to Pay More for Care, Poll Shows," *Trustee,* 1976, 29:4, 36.

6. E. R. Kingston and R. M. Scheffler, "Aging: Issues and Economic Trends for the 1980's," *Inquiry,* October 18, 1981, 18, 197-213. W. J. McNerny, "Control of Health Care Costs in the 1980's," *The New England Journal of Medicine,* November 6, 1980, 303:19, 1088-1095.

7. A. Donabedian, "Issues in National Health Insurance," *American Journal of Public Health,* 1976, 66:4, 345-350. *Health in the United States 1975: A Chartbook,* DHEW, Publication No. (HRA) 76-1233, 32.

8. M. S. Feldstein, *The Rising Cost of Hospital Care,* Washington, D.C.: Information Resources Press, 1971. E. F. X. Hughes, et al., "Surgical Workloads in a Community Practice," *Surgery,* 1972, 71:3, 315-325.

9. W. J. NcNerny, ibid, No. 6.

10. W. J. McNerny, ibid, No. 6. A. A. Scitovsky and N. McCall, "Coinsurance and the Demand for Physician Services: Four Years Later," *Social Security Bulletin,* 1977, 40:5, 19-27. J. P. Newhouse, *Insurance Benefits, Out-of-Pocket Payments, and the Demand for Medical Care: A Review of the Literature,* Santa Monica, California, The Rand Corporation, 1978.

11. M. Feldstein, *Hospital Costs and Health Insurance,* Cambridge, Harvard University Press, 1981. C. C. Havighurst, "Private Cost Containment Medical Practice Under Competition," in G. I. Misek (Ed.), *Socio Economic Issues of Health,* 1979, AMA, Monroe, Wisconsin, 1979, 41-66.

12. R. Fein, "Effects of Cost Sharing in Health Insurance: A Call for Caution," *The New England Journal of Medicine,* December 17, 1981, 305:25, 1526-1528.

13. L. Soderstrom, "The Canadian Experience," in A. Levin (Ed.), *Regulating Health Care,* New York, The Academy of Political Science, 1980, 33:4, 224-238. J. P. Geyman, "Reimbursement for Mental Health Services in Primary Care: Lessons from the Canadian Experience," *The Journal of Family Practice,* 13:6, 1981, 795-796. S. S. Lee, "Health Policy, A Social Contract: A Comparison of the United States and Canada," *Journal of Public Health Policy,* September, 1982, 293-301.

14. S. Sax, *Medicine in the 80's: Can We Afford It? The Australian Perspective,* The University of New South Wales School of Health Administration, Sydney, NSW, 1980.

15. J. P. Bunker, "Surgical Manpower: A Comparison of Operations and Surgeons in the United States, England and Wales," *The New England Journal of Medicine,* 1970, 282, 135-144.

16. Ibid, No. 15. G. S. Perrott, "The Federal Employees Health Benefits Program: Enrollment and Utilization of Health Services, 1961-68," US DHEW, HSMHA, Washington, D. C., 1971.

17. S. A. Schroeder, "Medical Technology and Academic Medicine: The Doctor-Producer's Dilemma," *Journal of Medical Education,* August 1981, 56, 634-639.

18. J. Showstack, S. A. Schroeder, and H. R. Steinberg, "Evaluating the Costs and Benefits of a Diagnostic Technology," *Medical Care,* May 1981, 19:5, 498-509.

19. "Interest in Primary Care Declines," *Socioeconomic Report,* California Medical Association, October/November 1981, 441:7, 2-5.

20. *Catastrophic Health Insurance,* Congressional Budget Office, Washington, D. C., U. S. Government Printing Office, 1977. *Minorities, Poverty and the Uninsured,* National Center for Health Services Research, Washington, D. C., 1981.

21. K. Davis, M. Gold, and D. Makuc, "Access to Health Care for the Poor: Does the Gap Remain?", *American Review of Public Health,* 1978, 2, 159-182. P.

W. Newacheck, et al., "Income and Illness," *MedicalCare,* 1980, 18:1, 1165-1176. "Minorities, Poverty and the Uninsured," National Center for Health Services Research, Publications and Information Branch Center Building, Room 7-44, 3700 East-West Highway, Hyattsville, Maryland, 20782.

22. H. L. Smitz, "Manpower for Long-Term Care: Two Simple Suggestions," in *Policy Forum, National Journal,* May 2, 1981, 807-809.

23. Towards a Comprehensive Health Policy, ibid, No. 3.

24. T. L. Delbanco, K. C. Meyers, and E. A. Segals, "Paying the Physician's Fee," *New England Journal of Medicine,* Dec. 13, 1979, 301:24, 1314-1320. L. Thomas, *The Lives of a Cell,* Bantam Books, Inc., New York, 1974, 35.

25. A. A. Scitovsky and N. McCall, "Changes in the Costs of Treatment of Selected Illnesses 1951-1964-1971," Health Policy Program, School of Medicine, University of California at San Francisco, August 1975.

26. *The Implications of Cost Effectiveness Analysis of Medical Technology,* Background Paper, No. 4: The Management of Health Care Technology in Ten Countries, OTA, Congress of the United States, Washington, D. C., October 1980, 3-8.

27. R. N. McKean, "Enforcement Costs in Environmental and Safety Regulation," *Policy Analysis,* Summer 1980, 6:3, 269-289. M. Pertschuk, *Revolt Against Regulation,* University of California Press, Berkeley, 1982, 137-156.

28. Lewin and Associates, Inc., *Evaluation of the Efficiency and Effectiveness of the Section 1122 Review Process, Parts I, II, III.* Washington, D. C., September 1975. W. B. Schwartz, "The Regulation Strategy for Controlling Hospital Costs," *The New England Journal of Medicine,* November 19, 1981, 305:21, 1249-1255. K. N. Lohr, J. D. Winkler, and R. H. Brook, *Peer Review and Technology Assessment in Medicine,* Santa Monica, Rand Publications, April 1976.

29. Ibid, No. 7. *Quality Assurance in Hospitals: Policy Alternative,* Boston, A. Springer International Publications, April 1976.

30. S. Law, *Blue Cross: What Went Wrong?,* Yale University Press, 1974, New Haven. Patrick O'Donoghue Policy Center, Inc., *Evidence About the Effects of Health Care Regulation,* Denver, Spectrum Research 1974, 45-58.

31. P. O'Donoghue, ibid, No. 30.

32. R. F. Knauss, "Health Manpower—The Right Kind," *Health Manpower Issues: A Presentation at the White House,* November 13, 1975, DHEW Publications (HRA) 76-40.

33. D. C. Williams, "Surgeons and Surgery in Rhode Island, 1970 and 1977," *New England Journal of Medicine,* Nov. 26, 1981, 305:22, 1319-1323. R. M. Scheffler et al, "A Manpower Policy for Primary Health Care," *New England Journal of Medicine,* May 11, 1978, 298, 1058-1062. R. M. Scheffler et al, "Physicians and New Health Practitioners: Issues for the 1980's," *Inquiry,* Fall, 1979, 16, 195-229. D. R. McNutt, "GMENAC: Its Manpower Forecasting Framework," *American Journal of Public Health,* Oct. 1981, 71:10, 1116-1124. U.E. Reinhardt, The GMENAC Forecast: An Alternative View," *American Journal of Public Health,* Oct. 1981, 71:10, 1149-1157.

34. Lewin and Associates, Inc., ibid, No. 28.

35. W. B. Schwartz, "The Regulation Strategy for Controlling Hospital Costs," *The New England Journal of Medicine,* November 19, 1981, 305:21, 1249-1255. R. G. Greene, D. Altman, and H. M. Sapolsky, *Health Planning and Regulation: The New England Experience,* Health Planning and Methods Technology Series, US DHHS, PHS, HRA HRP-0102201, March 1981. H. A. Foley, "Health Planning — Demise or Reformation?" *The New England Journal of Medicine,* April 16, 1981, 304:16, 969-972.

36. R. M. Battistella and S. R. Eastaugh, "Hospital Cost Containment," in A. Levin (Ed.), *Regulating Health Care,* New York, The Academy of Political Science, 1980, 33:4, 192-205.

37. D. Kinzer, "New Directions in Cost Containment," in *The Eye of the Beholder,* The Society for Health Policy Analysis, San Francisco, 1978, 11-15. Ibid, No. 13. "Rate Regulation," *Topics in Health Care Financing,* Fall 1979, 6:1, 1-139. P. O'Donoghue, ibid, No. 30.

38. *The Human Sized Hospital,* December 1981, 3:10, 1-6, AMI, Inc., 10390 Democracy Lane, Fairfax, Virginia 22030.

39. H. L. Smitz, "The PSRO in Perspective," *The New England Journal of Medicine,* July 30, 1981, 305:5, 253-259. Ibid, No. 27. R. G. Greene, et al., ibid, No. 35. Health Planning in Action, US DHHS, PHS HRA, HRP-0150201, August 1980.

40. *A Synthesis of Research on Competition in the Financing and Delivery of Health Services,* DHHS, Oct. 1982, Pub. No. (PHS) 83-3327. *Research on Competition in the Financing and Delivery of Health Services: Future Research Needs,* DHHS, Oct. 1982, Pub. No. (PHS) 83-3328-2. *Research on Competition in the Financing and Delivery of Health Services: A Summary of Policy Issues,* DHHS, Oct. 1982, Pub. No. (PHS) 83-3328-1.

41. C. E. Lindblom, *Politics and Markets,* New York, Basic Books, 1977.

42. M. S. Feldstein, ibid, No. 11. C. C. Havighurst, ibid, No. 11.

43. J. P. Newhouse, et al., "Some Interim Results from a Controlled Trial of Cost Sharing in Health Insurance," Santa Monica, Rand Publication Series R-2847-HHS, January 1982. Ibid, No. 10. Ibid, No. 11.

44. M. I. Roemer, et al., "Copayments for Ambulatory Care: Penny Wise and Pound Foolish," *Medical Care,* June 1975, XIII:6, 457-466. M. L. Barer, et al., "Controlling Health Costs by Direct Charges to Patients: Snare or Delusion?" Occasional Paper 10, Ontario, Canada, Ontario Economic Council, 1979.

45. A. C. Enthoven, *Health Plan,* Reading, Massachusetts, Addison Wesley, 1980. C. C. Havighurst, ibid, No. 11. M. S. Feldstein, ibid, No. 11. J. P. Newhouse, ibid, No. 10. R. Handschin, "Group Health Coop of Puget Sound," in Arizona Regional Medical Program Workshop on Alternative Methods for Delivery of Health Services, September 23-24, 1971, 43-55. H. S. Luft, *Health Maintenance Organizations,* New York, John Wiley and Sons, 1981. P. Ellwood, et al., "Health Maintenance Organizations: Concept and Strategy," *Hospitals,* March 16, 1971.

46. A. C. Enthoven, ibid, No. 45. P. Ellwood, ibid, No. 45.

47. E. Ginzberg, "Competition and Cost Containment," *The New England Journal of Medicine,* November 6, 1980, 303:19, 1112-1115. D. Neuhauser, "Enthoven's Health Plan," *The New England Journal of Medicine,* November

6, 1980, 303:19, 1115-1117. "Competition in the Health Care System: An Evaluation of the Pro-Competitive Bills," *Health Insurance Association of America,* March 1981.

48. A. C. Enthoven, ibid, No. 45. P. Caper, "Competition and Health Care, Caveat Emptor," *The New England Journal of Medicine,* May 21, 1981, 304:21, 1296-1299.

49. Ibid. No. 40. L. K. Ellwien and D. D. Gregg, "InterStudy Researchers Trace Progress of PPOs, Provides Insight Into Future Growth," *Federation of American Hospitals Review,* July/August '82, p. 20-25. "Health Care Industry, Business Show Increasing Interest in PPO Concept," *Federation of American Hosptials Review,* July/August '82, p. 12-18.

50. C. C. Havighurst, ibid, No. 11. C. C. Havighurst, "Antitrust Enforcement in the Medical Services Industry: What Does It All Mean?" *Milbank Memorial Fund Quarterly,* 58:1, 1980, 89-124.

51. L. B. Costello, "Competition, Policy and the Medical Profession," *The New England Journal of Medicine,* April 30, 1981, 304:18, 1099-1102.

52. W. J. Curran, "Health Planning, Blue Cross, and the Federal Antitrust Laws," *The New England Journal of Medicine,* November 12, 1981, 305:20, 1194-1195.

53. P. Feldstein, "The Political Environment of Regulation," in A. Levin (Ed.), *Regulating Health Care,* New York, The Academy of Political Science, 1980, 33:4, 6-20. U. E. Reinhardt, "Table Manners at the Health Care Feast," *Policy Forum, National Journal,* 5-11-81. M. R. Pollard, "Fostering Competition in Health Care," in *Regulating Health Care,* A. Levin (Ed.), New York, The Academy of Political Science, 1980, 158-167.

54. C. Wolf, Jr., *A Theory of Non-Market Failure,* Santa Monica, The Rand Corporation PG034, January 1978.

55. J. E. Affeldt, "The New Quality Assurance of the Joint Commission on Accreditation of Hospitals," *Western Journal of Medicine,* Feb. 1980, 132, 166-170.

56. C. E. Lindblom, ibid, No. 41.

57. J. Douglas, "Towards a Rationale for Private Non-Profit Organizations," PONPO Working Paper-7, Revised Version, New Haven, April 1980, Institution for Social and Policy Studies, Yale University. C. E. Lindblom, ibid, No. 56. R. Kramer, *Voluntary Agencies in the Welfare State,* Berkeley, University of California Press, 1981. J. Douglas and A. Wildavsky, "Big Government and the Private Foundations," *Policies Study Journal,* 1981, 9, 1175-1190.

58. A. L. Appelbaum, "The VE Gears Up for a Tough Year," *Trustee,* April 1979, 17-20.

59. "CVE," California Voluntary Health Care Cost Containment Effort, 1023-12th Street, Sacramento, California 95814, 1981.

60. "Enhancing Hospital Utilization Review," CVE, July 1981, California Voluntary Effort, Sacramento, California 95814.

61. H. L. Smitz, ibid, No. 39. H. N. Lohr, et al., ibid, No. 27. W. B. Schwartz, ibid, No. 27.

62. L. M. Salamon, "Rethinking Public Management," *Public Policy,* Summer 1981, 29:3, 255-275.

63. "Purchaser Health Care Cost Containment Initiatives," Western Center for Health Planning, San Francisco, October 1981. M. L. O'Connor, "Preferred Provider Organizations: A Market Approach to Health Care Competition" *Hospital Forum,* Nov.-Dec. 1982, 16-44.

64. R. F. Knauss, ibid, No. 32.

65. Health Characteristics by Geographic Region, Large Metropolitan Areas, and Other Places of Residence, NCHS, Series 10, No. 36, July 1963-June 1965, DHEW, PHS 1967. L. Montiero, "Expense is No Object: Income and Physician Visits Reconsidered," *Journal of Health and Social Behavior,* 1974, 14:2, 99-115. Ibid, No. 20. Ibid, No. 21. G. R. Wilensky and M. L. Berk, "The Health Care of the Poor and the Role of Medicaid," National Center for Health Sciences Research, Washington D.C., July 1982, Mimeo.

66. E. W. Hassinger, et al., "Changes in Number and Location of Health Practitioners in a 20-County Rural Area of Missouri," *Public Health Reports,* 1975, 90:4, 313-318. E. D. Martin, "The Federal Initiative in Rural Health," *Public Health Reports,* 1975, 90:4, 291-297.

67. K. Davis, "Equal Treatment and Unequal Benefits: The Medicare Program," *Milbank Memorial Fund Quarterly,* 1975, 53:4, 449-488. M. H. Ross, "Rural Health Care—Is Prepayment a Solution?" *Public Health Reports,* 1975, 90:4, 298-302. B. C. Stewart and L. A. Bair, *Health Care and Income (The Distributional Impacts of Medicaid and Medicare Nationally and in the State of Michigan),* Department of Social Services, State of Michigan, Lansing: Research Paper No. 5, April 1971.

68. E. D. Martin, ibid, No. 66. V. Navarro, "The Underdevelopment of Health in Rural America," paper presented at the *First National Conference on Rural America,* Washington, D.C., 1975, April 14-17. Towards a Comprehensive Health Policy, ibid, No. 3. H. U. Stambler, "Health Manpower—The Right Number," *Health Manpower Issues: A Presentation at the White House,* November 13, 1975, DHEW Publication (HRA) 76-40.

69. Minorities, etc., ibid, No. 21.

70. B. Spitz, "When a Solution is Not a Solution: Medicaid and Health Maintenance Organizations," *Journal of Health, Politics, Policy and Law,* Winter 1979, 3, 497-518.

71. E. D. Martin, ibid, No. 66. I. S. Moscovice and R. A. Rosenblatt, "Rural Health Care Delivery Amidst Federal Retrenchment: Lessons from the Robert Wood Johnson Foundation's Rural Project," *American Journal of Public Health,* Dec. 1981, 72:12, 1380-1385. D. Madison and C. Combs, "Location Patterns of Recent Physician Settlers in Rural America," *Journal of Community Health,* 1981, 6, 267-274. R. A. Rosenblatt, "Geographic Distribution of Board Certified Physicians," (Letters to the Editor) *New England Journal of Medicine,* 1981, 304, 916-917.

72. Interest in Primary Care, ibid, No. 19.

73. *Health in the U.S., 1975,* ibid, No. 7.

74. L. T. Barrett, "The Need for a Regional Focus in Rural Health Services," *Public Health Reports,* 1975, 90:4, 349-356. W. S. Beacham, "Appalachia, Testing Ground for Innovations," *Public Health Reports,* 1975, 90:4, 303-307.

75. D. A. Kindig, "Health Manpower—The Right Place," *Health Manpower Issues: A Presentation at the White House,* November 13, 1975, DHEW Publication (HRA) 76-40.

76. *World Development Report,* The World Bank, Washington, D.C., Aug. 1981, 175.

77. V. Navarro, ibid, No. 68.

78. A. Dickson, "Youth's Contribution to Health Care: Pediatrics in Reverse?" Commonwealth Secretariat Pre-World Health Assembly Meeting in Geneva, May 12, 1975, Marlborough House, Pall Mall, London, SW175HX. Institute of Medicine, *Community Oriented PrimaryCare,* Washington, D.C., National Academy Press, 1982.

79. J. P. Allegrante and L. W. Green, "When Health Policy Becomes Victim Blaming," *The New England Journal of Medicine,* December 17, 1981, 305:25, 1528-1529.

80. D. E. Hayes-Bautista, "Deviant Delivery Systems," prepared for Conference on National Health Policy, February 12 and 13, 1976, San Francisco, School of Public Health, University of California, Berkeley.

81. J. R. Bloom, "Models for Health Care Delivery," prepared for Conference on National Health Policy, February 12 and 13, 1976, San Francisco, School of Public Health, University of California, Berkeley.

82. N. A. Fuller, M. Patera and K. Koziol, "Medicaid Utilization of Services in a Prepaid Group Practice Plan," HMO Office, 5600 Fisher's Lane, Parklawn Building, Rockville, Maryland. C. R. Gaus, B. S. Cooper, and C. C. Hirschman, "Contrasts in HMO and Fee-for-Service Performance," Social Security Administration Office of Research and Statistics, Washington, D.C., 1976. R. Pineault, "The Effect of Prepaid Group Practice on Physician's Utilization Behavior," *MedicalCare,* 1976, 14:2, 121-136. C. J. Hynes, "The Regulation of Nursing Homes: A Case Study," in *Regulating HealthCare,* A. Levin (Ed.), New York, The Academy of Political Science, 33:4, 1980, 126-136.

83. R. M. Covell, "The Impact of Regulation on Health Care Quality," in A. Levin (Ed.), *Regulating Health Care,* New York, The Academy of Political Science, 1980, 33:4, 111-125.

84. A. Donabedian, "The Quality of Medical Care," in L. Carey, et al. (Eds.), *Medicine in a Changing Society,* St. Louis, C. V. Mosby, 1972, 83-101. A. Donabedian, "The Quality of Medical Care," in *Health United States 1978,* USDHEW, PHS 78-1232, Dec. 1978, 111-126.

85. R. P. Biller, "Disaggregating Health Promotion and Health Care: Policy Initiatives That Depend Less on Homogeneity Assumptions and More on Human Uniqueness," prepared for Conference on National Health Policy, February 12 and 13, 1976, San Francisco, Working Paper No. 49, Graduate School of Public Policy, University of California, Berkeley. D. Hayes-Bautista, ibid, No. 80.

86. H. L. Blum, "Evaluating Health Care," *MedicalCare,* December 1974, 12:12, 999-1011.

87. K. N. Lohr, et al., ibid, No. 27.

88. D. Hayes-Bautista, ibid, No. 80. J. M. Metsch and J. E. Veney, "Consumer Participation and Social Accountability," *MedicalCare,* 1976, 14:4, 283-293.

89. J. P. Allegrante, ibid, No. 79. K. G. Bauer, *Improving theChances for Health: Lifestyle Change and Health Evaluation,* National Center for Health Education, San Francisco, December 1980. N. Freudenberg, "Shaping the Future of Health Education: From Behavior Change to Social Change," *Health Education Monographs,* Winter 1978, 6:4, 372-376. N. Maccoby, et al., "Reducing the Risk of Cardiovascular Disease," *Journal ofCommunity Health,* Winter 1977, 3:2, 100-115.

90. L. Breslow and A. R. Somers, "The Lifetime Health-Monitoring Program," *The New England Journal of Medicine,* March 17, 1977, 296:11, 601-611.

91. C. E. Lewis, "Improving Access to Primary Care Through Reforms in Health Education, Orientations and Practice," in *Primary Care: Where Medicine Fails,* S. Andreopoulos (Ed.), New York, John Wiley and Sons, 1974, Chapter 2.

92. D. A. Kindig, ibid, No. 75. R. Kobernick, "WAMI, A Decentralized Medical Education Program in Washington, Alaska, Montana and Idaho," *Public Health Reports,* 1975, 90:4, 308-312. P. Rudd, "The United Farm Workers Clinic in Delano, California: A Study of the Rural Poor," *Public Health Reports,* July-August 1975, 90:4, 331-339.

93. L. Thomas, ibid, No. 24.

94. D. Mechanic, "Health and Illness in Technological Societies," *HastingsCenter Studies,* 1973, 1:3, 9-18.

95. M. Schaefer, *Intersectoral Coordination and Health in Environmental Management,* Geneva, WHO, Public Health Papers, 74, 1981.

96. K. L. White, "Health and Health Care: Personal and Public Issues," The 1974 Michael M. Davis Lecture, The Center for Health Administration Studies, Graduate School of Business, The University of Chicago.

97. Ibid, No. 13.

98. J. B. Christianson and W. McClure, "Incentives for Quality in a Restructured Medical Care System," *Policy Studies Journal,* 9:2, Special Issues. S. Jonas, "Planning for National Health Insurance by Objective: The Contract Mechanism," *Policy Studies Journal,* 9:2, Special Issues, No. 1, 1980-81, 250-259. D. B. Dutton, "Financial, Organizational, and Professional Determinants of Ambulatory Care and Implications for Medicaid Policy," mimeo paper, Health Services Research Division, Department of Family, Community, and Preventive Medicine, and Department of Sociology, Stanford University, Stanford, California, Sept. 16, 1982.

99. D. E. Beauchamp, "Public Health as Social Justice," *Inquiry,* 1976, 13, 3-14.

100. R. R. Alford, *Health Care Politics,* University of Chicago Press, Chicago, 1975.

Chapter 8

PLANNING AS A TOOL OF SOCIAL CHANGE

The processes that help us find our way from left to right on **Figure 1.1** (page **4**) (from philosophy about the "good" society and "good" health to relevant policy) are the task particularly of planners and policy analysts. These processes need not be intuitive. The steps and logics can be developed and learned. Although not explicitly presented, a planning approach took us from a reasonably-detailed examination of health to the services or processes that would be needed to maintain and improve health. In turn, if these processes were to be attained, we were shown that certain institutions and specially-trained personnel would be needed. And to attain these institutions, to keep them working in the ways called for, we were led to a national health policy that would foster and support these institutional forms while at the same time guaranteeing reasonable costs, equity of access to care, and improvement of health (our original philosophic or value base).

On **Figure 8.1**, we see the stages of planning for social change. The type of planning that we did in this book (essentially *normative* or *goal-based*) took our philosophy, values, and beliefs about "good" health and the "good" society (**Stage 1**) and turned them into a defined set of desired results (**Stage 10**), i.e., better health and health care for all at reasonable costs. We then worked "backward"deductively to establish the provider and client relationships and processes required (**Stage 9**). We next deduced the nature of service personnel, delivery units, and service programs (**Stages 8** and **7**) required to maintain the desired functional health-promoting roles and relationships of providers and clients. In turn, we deductively laid out the service agencies and systems (**Stages 6** and **5**) required to get us on the road to the desired results. Similarly deduced were the needed administration, guiding and enabling legislation, and policy (**Stages 4**, **3**, and **2**) to guide and provide for the subsequent **Stages 5-10**.

FIGURE 8.1

MOVING FROM ONE STAGE OF THE SOCIAL CHANGE SEQUENCE (SCS) TO THE NEXT: THE PLANNING PROCESS (PP) AS ENGINE* (Also see **FIGURE 8.2**)

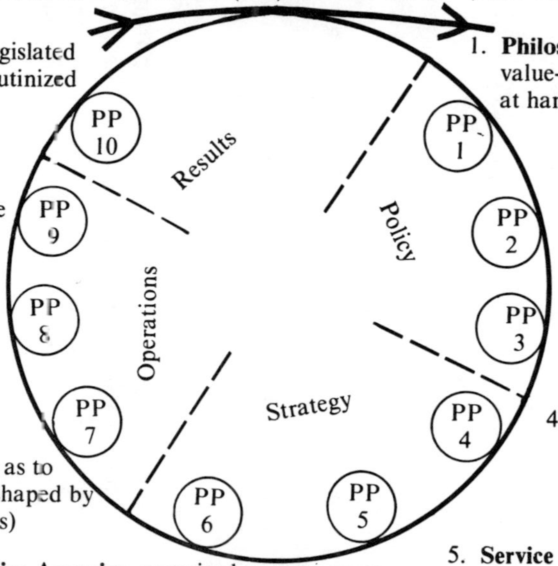

1. **Philosophy,** developed from implicit or explicit value-belief systems and applied to the concern at hand

2. **Policy,** formulated from philosophy (particularly the social-economic-political forces) as applied to the concern at hand

3. **Legislation,** formulated to carry out policy purposes (as shaped by personal and special interest concerns of legislators)

4. **Administration,** organized so as to carry out or oversee legislated purposes (as shaped by organizational and individual bureaucratic pressures)

5. **Service Systems,** organized so as to carry out legislated purposes (as shaped by pressures from established interests)

6. **Service Agencies,** organized so as to carry out legislated purposes (as shaped by pressures from currently viable units)

7. **Service Programs,** organized so as to achieve legislated purposes (as shaped by pressures from current providers)

8. **Service Delivery Units,** organized so as to carry out legislated purposes (as shaped by pressures from current providers-users)

9. **Server-Served Relationships,** built around personal role expectations and interactions called for by legislative mandate (as shaped by current provider-user pressures)

10. **Outcomes and impacts** of the legislated social change measured and scrutinized

*entire social change cycle and its stages shaped by the environmental force-field of cultures, traditions, values, beliefs, socio-economic-political ideologies, intra-national conflicts, political parties, governance, international pressures, and by the interests of those most involved at each stage.

Adapted from H. L. Blum, "Does Health Planning Work Anywhere?" *American Journal of Health Planning,* (July, 1978) 3:3, 34-47

Once it has become clear what all the stages call for, the major goals and needs are bundled into the policy, and legislation is written so that all the subsequent stages, in fact, will come to pass. Thus, the driving forces to obtain a desired social change are seen as the clockwise procession of **Stages 1** through **10**. In practice, in this form of planning, one first focused the philosophy, values, and beliefs, (**Stage 1**), so that the desired ends or results (**Stage 10**) stood out clearly. Having done that, one moves counter-clockwise from results, back along the cycle, so that when one returns to the level of policy (**Stage 2**), one sees fairly clearly what it must encompass. When policy is then converted into law (**Stage 3**), the latter needs to contain not only understanding of what is going to have to take place at the points of production, but the needed resources, constraints and enablements, and provide moral, as well as legal, guidance so that all the subsequent **Stages 4-9** will take place and give us the final results for which the SCS was intended. It turns out that this mode of planning has come to have a name of its own, **backward mapping.**[1]

There are many other approaches to planning, a good many of which will be presented in this chapter. In order to get a better grasp of what planning does encompass, we will pursue it somewhat generically. Planning for health or well-being, of necessity, has to be concerned with proposals for significant social changes, as well as for better delivery of health-promoting services by institutions which I believe must be quite differently oriented than most of those now available. How to determine what these should be accomplishing, what policy should be guiding them, and how they should be structured and operated, is what we expect from planning.

However, irrespective of one's beliefs in a general systems outlook on the origins of health, one conceivably might take any posture about what is to be done about social change and what are the tolerable or desirable means of achieving it. Such a posture quite justifiably even may be an aversion for any man-made conscious attempt, such as planning, to introduce social change.[2]

I. THE ORIGINS OF PLANNING

A. Purposes of Planning

The extensive literature on the purposes of planning provides many contrasting perspectives. Planning is variously described as being: an aid to or replacement of political decision making; a means of anticipating or looking ahead; a means of improving social justice; a means of improving the logic, science, or intellectual calibre of problem solving or reaching goals; the design efforts used to turn ideas into blueprints for action; the gentle persuasive route to getting equitable democratic decisions; and a means of control.[3]

I prefer a more prosaic view: we plan because we want change; we want change that represents "improvement." As a result, the planning process includes parts of all of the definitions presented. For me, planning has three major purposes: 1) **to define desired improvements**; 2) **to attain the desired improvements**; 3) **to evaluate the outcomes of the implemented planning.**

B. Origins of Desire for Change

The model of social change that I have found most helpful in understanding how demands for improvements result in social change has been described elsewhere.[4] Values lead to the setting of both goals and expectations (see **Figure 8.2**). Where expectations are not met, dissonance arises and causes a search for changes to meet the expectations and allay the dissonance. If there seems to be no hope of meeting the expectations, they may be lowered, goals may be changed, values may be altered, or the entire area suppressed from consciousness.

The model operates as follows:

1. Primal needs or natural drives, such as hunger, affection, or procreation, release and direct innate or primal energy to effectuate their satisfaction. Drives exist in a constantly shifting hierarchy, dependent in great part on how well each is satisfied at any given moment.

2. The overall environment determines how primal needs are best met and, as a result, valued behavior patterns and, subsequently, values emerge.

3. In each society the effective human interaction and survival behavior patterns have resulted in a well-structured value hierarchy even though innumerable sub-societal units have somewhat different hierarchies. New environmental demands and changes in sub-group behavior and intergroup relationships create a slow but constant shift in the hierarchy of values (valued behavior).

4. The innate energies available for meeting primal needs are transferred to the pursuit of values which, over time, may come to bear little more than symbolic relationships to the primal needs themselves. There is no evidence that the wellsprings of innate energy for achieving primal drives, now equally directed to achieving values and goals, ever dry up.

5. Because of the desire to reach certain achievements which fulfill these values, the values set corresponding goals and, thus, behavior.

6. A value also sets expectations or standards by which the value holder can decide whether the achievements, in fact, are adequate to reach the goals and satisfy the value.

FIGURE 8.2
VALUES AND CHANGE

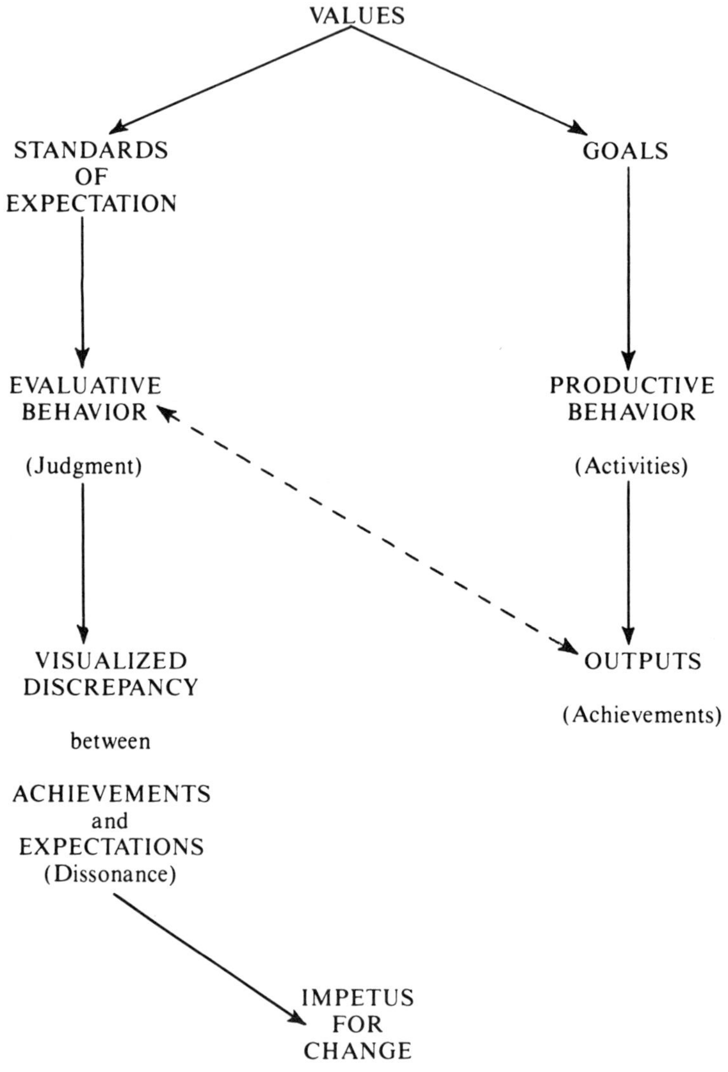

Adapted from H. L. Blum *Planning for Health*, Human Sciences Press, 2nd Edition, 1981, p. 46.

7. Discrepancies occur between what is perceived or believed to have been achieved in the way of reaching the desired goal set by a value and the standard of what is considered acceptable achievement as set up by the same value. The weighing of expectation versus accomplishment is done by individuals and groups.

Discrepancies also arise between values, or value systems, and role demands. Individual behavior is packaged into roles that must respond to many sub-sets of values and to many societal sub-systems. The many roles required of a person, therefore, are made congruent only with great difficulty.

8. With awareness of discrepancies, value holders come to feel the dissonance between achievement and expectation. Dissonance is intolerable to the value holder who therefore becomes desirous of change. Primal energies are released in amounts consonant with the degree of failure felt, and with the position of the unsatisfied value in the hierarchy of values.

9. Values also constitute the steering mechanism that guides the direction change will take.

10. Members of groups which have not yet learned or accepted the possibility or desirability of change respond to changes in their environment, or to dissonance from unsatisfied values, by expending more energy to avoid social change (which is a change of sorts) and maintain the status quo (i.e., negative feedback).

11. In change-oriented societies, the concept of being able to change has become acceptable as a way of responding to dissonance as well as to changes in environment and in the social system. (Significant change, not just the titillating variety, may even come to have a valued position in its own right.) Dissonance and change are expected to result in more social change (i.e., positive feedback), despite awareness that attempts to allay present strains or tensions will probably result in situations which produce new tensions.

12. To lower dissonance, individuals and societies commonly attempt, at least initially, to improve the performance of their activities or alter their environment so that current expectations and goals are met and values reasonably satisfied.

13. To lower dissonance, individuals and societies also may find it expedient to alter their goals, lower their norms for behavior or accomplishment, remodel or abandon unsatisfied values, or even adopt opposing ones.

14. There is no evidence that quieting dissonance by removing perceived discrepancies between achievement and expectation causes a cessation or necessarily even a long-term major slowdown in the evolution of new dissonances. The pace of growth and invention and their creation of new "needs" and environmental hazards, as well as the intellectual production of new vistas and new values, continues to alter the environment,

thereby setting the stage for dissonances produced by unsatisfied old values and the challenges to meet new ones.

15. There are four key determinants of social change;[5] the most important determinant is the **impetus** created by dissonance.

16. Three secondary determinants of the force and nature of social change are: 1) the structural or formalized social control setting; 2) informal social system pressures, or "self-regulation"; and 3) mobilization for change.

17. The energy exerted by the impetus for social change is directed heavily towards altering or revising the three secondary determinants in order to allow satisfaction of unsatisfied values or unacceptable role burdens or conflicts. As a result, changes in the three secondary determinants themselves may become the major, immediate, resultant social changes. These, in turn, become the instrumentalities from which a whole stream of other social changes may emerge.

No model can do justice to as complex a reality as societal functioning. But enough seems known about how an open system operates, and enough experience exists about planning as a means of introducing social change, that a model like this can serve as guidance to planners.

II. THE PLANNING PROCESS AS A MEANS OF IMPLEMENTING SOCIAL CHANGE

A. The Planning Process: a Cycle

The steps that are commonly described as constituting the cyclic planning process are outlined in **Figure 8.3.**

The arrows pointing clockwise indicate a theoretic flow of planning steps; each step leads to the next step by means of a specified activity.

No one step is individually identified with any one of the three major planning purposes. However, **Steps a** and **b** relate particularly to the purpose of discovering, defining, and prioritizing wanted improvements (in the form of goals to be reached and/or of current problems to be remedied). **Steps c** and **d** take planning through the analytic and design phases, while **e** encompasses the political and action implementation stages to achieve the second purpose of planning, i.e., bring the wanted improvements to fruition. **Step f**, the evaluation phase, serves the third major purpose of planning, which is to see what planning has produced and how well it has succeeded. (The major uses of evaluation in this context are

FIGURE 8.3
ELEMENTS OF THE PLANNING PROCESS (PP)*

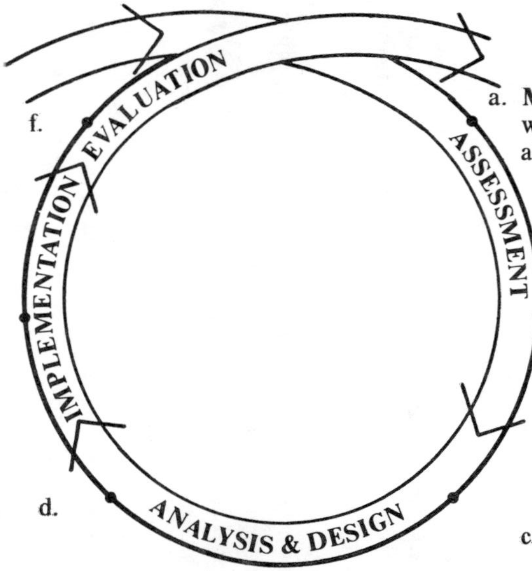

a. **Measurement,** determination of where we are, where we are likely to be, how we feel about it, and what we want

b. **Interpretation of data,** identification and selection of wants (problems or goals) and grand ideologic **GOALS**

c. **Analysis,** understanding nature of specific wants

d. **Creating the plan,** design, analysis, comparison, and selection among alternative interventions.

e. **Implementation,** obtaining policy commitment and bureaucratic action on the plan

f. **Evaluation,** analyzing the outputs, outcomes, and impacts occurring as a result of planning

*entire process and elements guided by the prevalent socio-economic-political outlooks, relevant legislated policies, political environment, resources, governmental structure, and planning expertise

Adapted from H. L. Blum, "Does Planning Work Anywhere?" *American Journal of Health Planning,* (July, 1978) 3:3, 34-47 to gain understanding about the nature of the systems being affected, the quality of the planning, the nature of the outcomes, the continued desirability of the goals, and how to redirect future planning in the light of such knowledge.) It is important to recognize that each planning step also carries evaluative possibilities about prior steps, and that one dare not overlook these early evaluative opportunities.

B. The Social Change Sequence: Implementation

Implementation is the only legitimate reason for undertaking planning to produce change. True, we are all aware that much of planning is undertaken to forestall action and to avoid introducing significant change. We in the U.S. also are well aware that national health planning policy, as expressed in P. L.89-749, of 1966, explicitly forbade contemplation of change in the mode of health care delivery, i.e., its "Findings and Declaration of Purpose" conclude with the phrase, *without interference with existing patterns of private professional practice of medicine, dentistry, and related healing arts.*

Figure 8.1 tries to make clear what implementation consists of for any significant proposed social change. It involves making every stage of the effort explicit, and finding the way to achieve the planned product.

At **Stage 1**, the planners will be involved in articulating and striking compromises among the dominant or significant philosophies so that a coherent approach is promulgated.

For **Stage 2**, planners will be designing a policy that makes the philosophy adequately explicit so that it can be used as specific guidance for checking any plans or proposals in the area of concern.

For **Stage 3**, they will be designing the legislation and "greasing the legislative machinery" so that the policy becomes law and carries with it enough resources, stated purposes, suitable machinery, and controls or incentives so that the subsequent stages of the cycle can and will take place.

For **Stage 4**, the planners design the top-level controlling and enabling administrative mechanism that will want to carry out the legislation, and that is capable, as well as desirous, of providing the relevant guidance for the service systems and all subsequent levels that take over the key **doing** tasks.

For **Stage 5**, the planners design service systems or organizational networks that are capable and desirous of creating and supporting the service agencies envisioned as carrying out the needed tasks.

For **Stage 6**, the planners design the service agencies that are capable and desirous of operating the envisioned actual delivery entities.

For **Stage 7**, the planners design the service delivery programs that are capable and desirous of creating needed delivery units.

For **Stage 8**, the planners design the service delivery units that can support the provider-client relationships and utilization of services that were foreseen as necessary.

For **Stage 9**, the planners design the client-provider relationships that encourage and bring about client and provider roles that will result in better health.

For **Stage 10**, the planners design ways of measuring work output, outcomes to those served, and impacts on the larger society.

At the beginning of this chapter, it was pointed out that the form of planning used in this book involved the deductive steps of working counter-clockwise from the desired results. However, putting the machinery into operation then involves starting at the beginning of the cycle, and laying out the means of going step-by-step clockwise around the cycle, so that what was deduced in a counter-clockwise order comes to pass in the necessary clockwise order.

C. Applying the Planning Process Cycle to the Social Change Sequence

Now we must examine how the Planning Process cycle (PP) steps relate to the Social Change Sequence (SCS). The PP is repeated at each stage of the SCS. Although the substrate of what is to be acted on by the planning elements varies at each stage of the SCS, the elements of the planning cycle used at each stage are not remarkably different.

Figure 8.1 showed how the two cycles interrelate: the PP one being the small drive wheel at each stage that moves the larger change (SCS) wheel.

In common parlance, those who concentrate on the planning process at the first three stages of the SCS are likely to be called **policy planners** or **analysts**. True, their concerns also include, at a lesser level of detail, all subsequent stages and actors of the SCS under consideration, whether it be health care, environmental protection, or whatever.

Of critical interest to these policy planners is how to get their handiwork implemented into law. They must determine who will help and who will hinder, and how to harness the favorable and overcome the hostile forces. And since implementation means that the planners must extend their sights on down the SCS, they must have decided how, in fact, the jobs called for by the subsequent stages will get done, as each stage is responsible for its own tasks as well as for the suitable functioning of all the subsequent stages.

If we take an example of a health care social change instigated at the Federal level, there are numerous options for getting meaningful compliance with the policy. (See **Figure 7.2**, page **187**.) The Federal government could produce the services itself, as it does in the V.A. Alternatively, it could exert explicit and total control over private for-profit or non-profit operational entities, treating them as public utilities. It could work by contracting for services with public or private for-profit or non-profit producers, as it does with Medicare. It could organize its services by handing them off to states (as it does with Medicaid), which, in turn, may further hand them off to private for-profit and non-profit entities, or to local governments, on a fee-for-service or per-capitation basis. As suggested in the policy chapter (7) of this book, government could be a finance collecting and redistributing mechanism which removes all government levels from current types of service production, and, at the same time, so constrain the market as to put all citizens into a comprehensive Health Care Delivery System of their own choice. President Reagan envisioned a further development in which the Federal government neither finances, redistributes, nor produces any services; instead, turning all persons, including the impoverished, over to the production vagaries of our unfettered market place that supplies to those with purchasing power what they wish to buy.

Those who concentrate on the planning process cycling at **Stages 4-6** of the SCS are often called **strategic**, **programmatic**, or **systems planners**. They have responsibility for all the subsequent stages of the SCS as well, although at a lesser level of detail.

Those whose primary concern is with planning at **Stages 7-9** of the SCS are the **administrators** (administrative planners), who convert the inputs into processes and activities that cause the wanted results to occur.

At every level, results or evidences of accomplishment are counted and fed back up to the policy level. The policy-level people must also be the ones who look for evidence of unexpected favorable and unfavorable impacts on society of the measured outputs and outcomes. A much more elaborate and realistic look at this whole operation is available.[6] It shows how socio-economic-political outlook, form of governance, stage of development and resource availability, gifts and constraints from other levels of government or from other societies, cultural outlooks, and so on, all affect both the possibilities for planning and the forms that it can take.

III. ALTERNATIVE MODES OF PLANNING

A. Eight Common Prototypes

There are scores of described modes of planning.[7] They tend to be distinguished by their emphasis on one or another consideration, such as key roles to be served by the process, nature of control, participation in the process, degree of future orientation, boundaries, the extent to which values are promoted, and so on. One attempt to sort them out has been to create a typology of planning bodies in accordance with their sources and extent of authority.[8]

The eight modes to be described here emphasize how extensive and critical the differences are between different approaches to planning for the achievement of social change. The critical point to be made is that each mode is very likely to lead to different plans and outcomes. In fact, each mode incorporates assumptions and technologies based on different value hierarchies.

Figure 8.4 presents a spectrum of representative planning outlooks relevant to health planning. Reading from **1** to **8**, the modes imply a generally increasing intent to intervene, and an increasing complexity consistent with their increasing intent to deal with the interrelatedness of all aspects of living. The vertical columns provide a brief description of the characteristics of each mode, and a few additional words about each will further illustrate their differences and utilities.

Laissez-faire contrasted with total planning **Laissez-faire** in planning, the exact extreme of the **total planning** approach, refers to the intentional neglect of planning in favor of the use of the principles of the free market and purchasing power to achieve society's goals. It can be demonstrated, however, that purchasing power is a highly-partial force that will find few of the poor receiving care and few using preventive services. The environment of the transactions in the market must be rigged nowadays by critical, major, planned policies, if we are to achieve such crucial social (non-market) goals as equity of distribution of services to the poor or the isolated. Examples of such publicly-arranged rigging are special taxes, bonuses, subsidies, depletion allowances, quotas, and tax write-offs, so that even if there is a market it is driven to operate in limited or directed ways.

By contrast, if each of the presently-occurring market transactions were to be planned and programmed, we would enter the ordered future of total planning, which also has no brilliant record for coming out where desired. It is not clear, either, that "total" planning for the health sector is even possible unless the entire economy is also totally planned. Conformance of every unit of health care service to some pre-specified blueprint would simultaneously put constraints on every other use of resources, even on the overt acts permitted. As a further objection to total planning, we point out that the obsession with specification of detail has long been known to engender enforcement for its own sake, irrespective of whether it facilitates reaching major goals or solving major problems.

The appeal of total planning and the avoidance of laissez-faire obviously must lie in another direction. Total planning is more often seen as applicable in a society where a well-developed dogma or credo has been turned into a full set of widely-accepted or rigorously-indoctrinated goals, which have been converted, in turn, into strategies, methods, and tools that

FIGURE 8.4
A COMPARISON OF PLANNING MODES

	PRESENT OR SHORT-RANGE CONCERNS			
	1. Laissez-faire	2. Disjointed incrementalism, problem amelioration	3. Allocative	4. Articulated and guided incrementalism, problem solving
	No planning	Minimal planning	Minimal planning for the present or near future	Planning for the present or near future
Planning mode	Leave market unfettered and eliminate need for public programs, private planning unfettered	Apply obvious remedies to undesirable situations as they become intolerable	Allocate resources in accordance with evidence of effectivity of current programs and meet high-priority new problems	Analyze problems in terms of system in which they are embedded and design interventions accordingly, select for implementation according to larger societal goals
"Present" or short-range results	Problems will disappear	Ameliorate present problems	Alter priorities and present problems	Ameloriate present problems and future ones

	MIDDLE AND LONG-RANGE CONCERNS			
	5. Exploitive	6. Explorative	7. normative	8. Total planning
	Planning with the future	Planning towards the future	Planning from the future	Planning for all activities, present and future
Planning mode	Determine and make the most of trends and allocate resources so as to take advantage of what is to come	Explore the futures possible from current trends, capacities, expectations, and design a desired[2] feasible future. Allocate resources accordingly	Decide on the future desired[3] and allocate resource so that programs and trends are created accordingly	Decide on the future and present desired, and lay out use of all resources accordingly
"Present" or short-range results	A sense of triumphing over fear. Take advantage of what is coming	A sense of choosing the best feasible destiny. Seek what could be	A sense of helping create destiny. Seek what should be	A sense of controlling all destinies

[1]Adapted from R. Kaje, personal communication
[2]Usually done on a basis of current or predicted values
[3]Can be done on a basis of current values, predicted values, or creating new values

Adapted from H. L. Blum, *Planning for Health*, New York Human Sciences Press, 1974, p. 56-59.

presumably guarantee goal-envisioned outcomes.

Societies that accept pluralistic views are less sure of their ability to designate all-encompassing goals, or to design interventions that will unfailingly reach them. They are more likely to operate on a majority consensus open to frequent alteration, or even to the possibility of peaceful major reversals. Truly pluralistic societies encourage or tolerate many diverse goals, and conflicting ones are not quarantined officially in an attempt to reach one over-riding set. The more open societies, particularly those where there is a wide dispersion of power, never could agree then on a solid phalanx of goals, and therefore could never use total planning. By the same token, pluralistic societies use incentives and "rigging" of the market place in their planning, while preserving as much laissez-faire for the daily small acts as possible.

In our society laissez-faire has come to mean that there shall be no formal, visible planning on behalf of the public by government. It does mean private planning for private gain on a monumental scale because of the size and long-term commitments that must be made in the vast, corporate, technological undertakings that create our society's productivity. Unfortunately, private gain is not necessarily synonymous with the well-being of the public. Even where there are millions of shareholders in a private enterprise, their interests focus on the returns or the direct value of their shares, and not on corporate directions that may use the whole world's supply of energy wastefully, create inefficient and dangerous modes of transport, or poison such precious resources as air, water, and soil. There is little likelihood that widely-participative ownership in private concerns can convert planning for private gain into planning for public good.

Disjointed incrementalism, contrasted with articulated and guided incrementalism The most accepted model for pursuing deliberate social change in the U.S. is named, appropriately, **Disjointed Incrementalism**. Braybrooke and Lindblom argued that decision makers in a democracy like the U.S. do and should use a pragmatic approach that involves making relatively small improvements based on a comparison of a limited number of alternative proposals.[9] The arguments for the approach are:

- the lack of comprehensive information available to decision makers
- man's limited problem-solving capabilities
- the unlimited nature of alternatives
- the costliness of comprehensive analysis
- the inability of planners to construct a satisfactory method of evaluating values or goals

- the openness of any system to the fluidity and range of variables that have to be dealt with
- the inability of administrators to intelligently evaluate the consequences of interventions
- the utility of small steps, the repercussions of which serve to guide us
- the multiple bases from which separate, small decisions must be seen and, in fact, are made, and the consequent inability of each base to look at more than a small fragment of an issue
- the multiplicity of decision-making bases which, in the aggregate, provide reasonable coverage

Disjointed incrementalism is designed to respond to felt hurts (i.e., problems) in a fairly-rapid way. It primarily seeks to allay what can no longer be put off. It is built on a philosophy of active growth, unlimited opportunity, and minimal design, limited to "greasing the squeaky wheel" without affecting or restraining too much else. Its greatest failures lie in the damage such short-run and poorly-conceived corrections seem to produce, and in the subsequent need for additional, similarly blindly-concocted, patches on top of patches. In a critical revision of their thinking, Dahl and Lindblom part sharply with their visions of success by pluralistic, disjointed-incrementalistic bargaining, and state that *The new problems, it may turn out, are problems for all of us: their prototypes are energy depletion, environmental degradation, and the gap between the advanced and developing nations.*[10]

By contrast, then, many believe that **Guided and Articulated Incrementalism**, also reserved for correction of problems, has more to offer. Guided and articulated incrementalism begins with guidance from the long-range, over-arching goals society proclaims for itself (see **Normative Planning**, page **224**). Planning is begun with an acknowledgment of such goals, even if the intent is to give priority to current problems.

Guidance from major societal goals is required if incrementalism is to be free from the hazards of problem-solutions that violate, move away from, or obstruct attainment of cherished societal goals. In this way, long-term goals guide the planners through problem solving so that remedies for problems do not set up long-term incompatabilities with goals.

Articulation speaks to the need to understand the forces at work in the system in which the problem occurs, so that possible points of attack on the problem are revealed and the major parties at interest identified. Careful scrutiny is given to the multiple points at which attack is possible, to multiple modes of intervention possible at each point, and to the desirability of combinations of such interventions. Each proposed solution, which may be a package of interventions, is subjected to a reasonable study of the probable nature and extent of the good it will do (benefits), and of its costs, which include the probable direct costs of carrying it out, and the undesired outcomes it may create in one way or another. One well-developed example illustrates the benefit and cost possibilities from alternative attacks on tuberculosis.[11] There is an excellent collection of not-so-well-developed interventions for various problems that resulted in wholesale disasters.[12] The probable gains and losses, and to whom they will occur, have been examined for such large issues as legalized gambling[13] and accountability in education.[14] The issues of gains and losses from transfers in an urbanized economy recently have been examined in many contexts.[15] This area of weighing alternative interventions is considered to be the field of policy analysis as well as of planning.[16]

Guided and articulated incrementalism does not seem beyond our grasp. Attempts to use it are unlikely to harm us as much as the "harum-scarum" cosmetic patches resulting from disjointed incrementalism.

Allocative planning The major justification for **allocative planning**, which is designed to get the most from each dollar invested, is in making shifts away from programs considered to be less profitable toward those with a presumably higher payoff. This mode of planning is particularly useful at the time of making resource allocation decisions among the activities in a given program, area, or sector, when the majority of the problems involved and the activities directed at them cannot be analyzed carefully in any one budget period.

The weakness of this mode is its general unconcern for goals. Its economic, cost-benefit outlook is likely to lead it to the "best buys" in dollar or production terms, and ignore less economically-measurable outcomes, or abandon programs that deal with such less-productive persons as the aged, poor, children, or minorities.

Exploitive planning The wise use of exploitive planning, which depends on creditable prognostications as to what will come to pass, is of use in getting "piggy-back" rides from time to time, e.g., certain undesired conditions can be foreseen as melting away by themselves, or goals can be seen as being approached or facilitated by inevitable, even if unintended, results of other streams of ongoing activities. With such insights, various programs or expenditures can be avoided, and the same resources can be put into other areas where high-priority goals otherwise would not be achieved without new investment. Similarly, foreseen developments allow planners to build further extensions or speed up the process if it is desired.

The weakness of this mode is its common unconcern for undesirable futures or how to avoid them. Rather, it is likely to accept a highly-probable given future, even promote it if a profit can be turned, in spite of a high probability of an overall undesirable outcome once a way has been found to exploit it.

Normative and explorative planning, complementary and contrasting The quickest summation of what distinguishes **normative planning** from all the others is its stipulation of what we believe **ought to be**. Normative planners have three options: a) they may use present-day values as guides to the ideal; b) they may try to prognosticate the values and the ideals that will be prevalent at the time the product of planning is emerging; c) finally, they may build a whole new set of values that will shape the future they want. It is the latter "willed" future of Ozbekhan that gives rise to great religious and political movements, such as the creation of the U.S. or of the Soviet Union and their new forms of government.[17] All the normative modes require the planner to work back from the chosen goals to the changes which must be implemented today and tomorrow if the long-range goals are to be reached.

Explorative planning establishes a picture of the future by studying extensions of capacities, desires, and possibilities from the viewpoint of what the present offers. It represents an extension of the present, even though extensions may be bent by what is currently wanted, but not presently available, so that the future is not merely an extension of the present but an extension of what study of the present indicates *could be*. Explorative planning sets up long-term possible goals out of the forecasts of what could be. The fact that acceptance of possible goals means that they also must be desirable ones makes explorative planning somewhat normative. But it differs from normative planning, which starts with a determination of what present or future values *would* call for, or even with a "willed future" which starts by a break with current values and postulates new values as to what ought to be.

Normative and explorative modes intertwine, of necessity. A beginning from either promptly leads to elements of the other. A normative declaration promptly requires an exploratory thrust to determine what is possible. An exploratory declaration of what is possible promptly leads to a normative formulation of what is desirable.[18]

B. Developmental Planning as the Mode of Choice

The developmental approach to planning combines normative planning (goal attainment) with guided and articulated planning (problem solving).[19] In other words, in addition to defining major goals and planning to reach them, it uses the same goals as a source of guidance for problem solving. Thus, current problems are addressed by solutions that are designed to be compatible with desired large-goal directions.

The proposals in this book are based on a set of goals that are clearly normative, but they also offer many articulated and guided changes which are incremental. In actual practice, few societies not undergoing revolution would try to institute a whole new system without building on the usable elements currently available, and without attempting correction of the worst messes in current services. Similar mixed planning approaches have been advocated previously, as "middle range bridge,"[20] and "mixed scanning."[21]

Developmental planning strives to reach formulated goals, both directly and incrementally. How heavily it uses one or the other of the approaches varies in accordance with the nature of the situation and the political outlook of the community. Placing a man on the moon was done all of a piece. Correction of our inadequate health status and of the medical care mess in the ways I believe are needed, unless handled in an equally normative way, apparently will take even more decades of public intervention than those behind us.

Because of its overwhelming dependence on all other aspects of our life, and on the behavior of people and institutions, major changes in content or form of health care delivery are hard to agree on politically, even when there is agreement on goals. Developmental planning proposes that we establish goals for health. Some of these goals can be planned directly. At the same time, continuing evaluation tells us how well we are approaching these long-range goals. We alter our plans (perhaps even our goals) by what we learn about the outcomes occurring from our current interventions.

Developmental planning is quite eclectic. Although it avoids total planning and disjointed incrementalism assiduously, it utilizes many other approaches to planning in addition to the normative and the articulated and guided incremental modes. It uses exploratory planning to probe the future. It accepts the utility of allocative planning for the large areas of policy decision which cannot be reviewed every year, or which cannot be addressed economically by the planning currently underway. It is anxious to utilize exploitive planning to the degree that it supplies foresight and provides evidences of "free" successes that are about to occur without planning effort, but which are consistent with established goals.

Laissez-faire, the imperfect capitalist market place so well-known to us, would continue as the means of making nearly all transactions. However, in contrast to the present deformation of the market by powerful private forces and by innumerable and poorly-developed, politically-expedient, public forces, the market would be guided and constrained by public policies derived from the normative goals generally accepted for the country. Such a market was envisioned in **Chapter 7**.

Thus, developmental planning tries to utilize a society's value system as guidance for the long-range and the short-range planning efforts. Politically it seems impossible and morally it seems unacceptable to avoid correcting present hurts. Rationally and humanistically, it seems indefensible not to try to approach goals which are highly-desired generally, such as peace, freedom from want, or better health. Developmental planning tries to bring these short- and long-term purposes together.

IV. IMPROVEMENT FOR WHOM?

The key planning question always revolves around "improvement for whom?" There seems to be no alternative but to involve all of the relevant diversity of interests in the planning, as well as in the operation of what has been planned. In particular, those whom society currently labels as deviant (sick, criminal, addicted, dropout, etc.) must be present in the goal setting, problem analysis, design of interventions, and implementation of the very system which has labeled them deviant (health, justice, education, etc.), and which is trying to "help" them. This is an essential, countervailing device for planning and policy making if we really care about whose improvement we are proposing, the nature of that improvement, and the likelihood that anything desired will happen. Even though we may all share similar goals, it is not sensible to place today's non-deviants and professionals, who are trained to track down and treat deviants, in exclusive charge of deciding what "improvements" consist of or how they are to be obtained. Society labels the deviant, no matter whether its intent is restoration, constraint, or punishment. It is time for society to accept the fact that it is being modified by the pressure of the deviant, and by its acknowledgment of, and by its behavior to, deviants. If society is to add to its comprehension of the forces at work in creating deviancy and social change, and to its capacity for changing appropriately in response to new forces, it must do better than to blindly ignore the deviant point of view.

V. PERSONAL AGENDAS DETERMINE PLANNED-FOR ENDS AND PLANNING MEANS

My major overall health objective might be described as "better health." My major social objectives can be described as creating maximum participation or opportunity for determination of health goals, and for awareness of the possibilities of how to reach them. These sets of objectives, in turn, have been created by my major social values, which are: **participatory decision making, maximal personal liberty and choice within a legal framework**, **equality of opportunity**, and **equity in access to well-being services**. From among several options, I have chosen to give the term **equity** the meaning of "fairness and availability of services in accordance with well-being needs," rather than in accordance with such a factor as purchasing power.[22]

If the systems concept of the nature of health (**Chapter 2**) and my goal of better health are accepted, but my value of equity or my beliefs about human nature and the necessity for participative democracy are not, other planned approaches to a better state of health can be suggested by those holding such views and applying them to the *homo sapiens* hierarchy of systems.[23]

My professionally-biased value configuration has led me to adopt the developmental planning mode. In turn, developmental planning has led me to make several proposals in the prior chapters about how to improve health inside such a value framework. If these views strike a responsive chord, they, and innumerable modifications, or perhaps quite-different but equally-relevant proposals, may suggest themselves to the reader as being more acceptable.

For those who oppose public interventions into any area where a profit can be made, public planning and legislating for health care are not acceptable. For those who do not, or cannot, believe in our capacity to plan, or in the long-range utility of trying to nudge ecology in a way favorable to health, planning for significant changes in health care is useless.

By way of conclusion about the scope of planning and its response to values, this is a good time to return to our concept of the systems hierarchy of *homo sapiens,* as illustrated in **Figure 2.1**, page **7**. Let us remind ourselves that the significant perturbations in and among the various levels of systems become ill-health. It is therefore fascinating to observe that many planners tend to concentrate on designing interventions for one or another level of system.[24] The so-called radicals of the left, such as Navarro[25] and Congressman Dellums, and those on the right, such as Milton Friedman and President Reagan, constantly call our attention to options which have as their goal the revising of our cultural beliefs and values; which in turn, of course, call for new forms of societal organization. This is an attack very high up on our hierarchy.

Other planners tend to gravitate to the lower levels of societal systems, and suggest juggling the sectors and their institutions. Enthoven[26] and Martin Feldstein[27] provide prominent examples of such interveners.

Some "planners" tend to work at still lower levels and direct their efforts to patching the delivery machinery to make it more efficient, more responsive, or less costly. Prominent among these persons are Walter McNerny[28] and Harold Luft.[29]

Some "planners" tend to work at the level of the family and social networks. Persons such as Leonard Syme[30] are well known in this area.

Other "planners," such as Farquhar et al.,[31] tend to work predominantly on the individual and behavior modifications. Their work is commonly called **risk reduction**.

Still other "planners," identified heavily with the so-called medical or sickness model, work with the systems levels incorporated beneath, or inside, the person level. Every medical center and school has its eminent biologic "health" planners at work, designing methods to understand the sub-organic and organic systems and to overcome their perturbations. In some medically-based institutions there has been a heavy extension of interest to sickness-proofing various of the person's sub-systems, i.e., doing preventive medicine. Persons such as Jonathan Fielding are well-known in this area.[32]

By no means would I imply that the above named individuals only work at one or another level of systems, but it is clear that some of their best-known work is directed at certain levels, primarily.

A few of us, who see the planning process and implementation of goals as our central work, attempt to take into account any or all of the levels all of the time; and I would make a plea that planners do a suitable analysis or examination of each issue so that it becomes clear which systems levels hold possibilities for intervention.[33] To a great extent, it is true that each issue has to be taken to that system level where a satisfying solution is feasible. It is also true that one or more solutions for a given issue may exist at many systems levels. A fairly simple example is that of injuries due to accidents at unguarded railroad-highway crossings. At one level of system, these call for extensive emergency services of many kinds, including direct medical repair, to be followed by rehabilitation and maintenance of handicapped victims. At another level, it is possible to work on the education of individuals to make them more alert to, and able to avoid, hazards at such crossings. At still another level, it is possible likewise to make the crossings less hazardous by installation of warnings, etc. It is also possible to intervene at the higher system level of social legislation, so that all such traffic crossings must separate the two transport schemes by overhead or underground crossings.

Hopefully, our planners will examine possibilities for intervention at all systems levels, and then help us decide which best suit our values, our pocketbook, and our health needs.

REFERENCES

1. R. F. Elmore, "Backward Mapping: Implementation Research and Policy Decisions," *Political Science Quarterly,* Winter 1979-80, 94:4, 601-615. R. F. Elmore, *Complexity and Control: What Legislators and Administrators Can Do About Implementing Public Policy,* U.S. Department of Education, National Institute of Education, Washington, D.C., August 1980.

2. A. Wildavsky, "If Planning is Everything, Maybe It's Nothing," *Policy Sciences,* 4, 1973, 125-33. F. A. Hayek, *The Road to Serfdom,* Chicago, Chicago University Press, 1944.

3. H. L. Blum, *Planning for Health,* 2nd Edition, New York, Human Sciences Press, 1981, 72-74.

4. H. L. Blum, ibid, No. 3, 39-80.

5. N. J. Smelser, "Toward a General Theory of Social Change," *Essays in Sociological Explanation,* N. J. Smelser (Ed.), Englewood Cliffs, New Jersey, Prentice-Hall, Inc. 1968. 205.

6. H. L. Blum, ibid, No. 3, 56-70.

7. H. L. Blum, ibid, No. 3, 319-323.

8. H. H. Hyman, *Health Planning: A Systematic Approach,* Germantown, Maryland, Aspen Systems Corporation, 1976.

9. D. Braybrooke and C. E. Lindblom, *A Strategy for Decision,* New York, The Free Press, 1963.

10. R. A. Dahl and C. E. Lindblom, *Politics, Economics and Welfare,* 2nd Edition, New York, Harper and Row, 1976, Preface, 1976, XXII.

11. M. S. Feldstein, M.A. Piot, and T. K. Sundaresan, "Resource Allocation Model for Public Health Planning—A Case Study for Tuberculosis Control," Supplement to Volume 48 of the Bulletin of the World Health Organization, Geneva, WHO, 1973.

12. T. Farvor and J. Milton, *Careless Technology,* New York, Natural History Press, 1972.

13. J. Marcum and H. Rowen, "How Many Games in Town? The Pros and Cons of Legalized Gambling," *The Public Interest,* 1974, 36: 25-52.

14. J. T. Murphy and D. K. Cohne, "Accountability in Education: The Michigan Experience," *The Public Interest,* 1974, 36: 53-81.

15. K. E. Boulding, M. Pfaff and A. Pfaff, *Transfers in an Urbanized Economy,* Belmont, California, Wadsworth Publishing Company, 1973.

16. C. E. Lindblom, *The Policy Making Process,* Englewood Cliffs, New Jersey, 1968, Chapters 2, 3, 4.

17. H. Ozbekhan, "Towards a General Theory of Planning," in *Perspectives in Planning,* E. Jantsch (Ed.), Paris, Organization for Economic Cooperation and Development, 1969, 47-159.

18. E. Jantsch, *Technological Forecasting in Perspective,* Paris, Organization for Economic Cooperation and Development, 1967, Chapters 1 and 2.

19. H. L. Blum, ibid, No. 3, 80-81.

20. M. Meyerson, "Building the Middle Range Bridge for Comprehensive Planning," *Journal of the American Institute of Planners,* 1956, 22: 58-64.

21. A. Etzioni, *The Active Society.* New York, The Free Press, Chapter 12.

22. N. Gilbert and H. Specht, *Dimensions of Social Welfare Policy,* Englewood Cliffs, New Jersey, Prentice Hall Inc., 1974, 40-41.

23. C. W. Churchman, *Challenge to Reason,* New York, McGraw-Hill, 1968. C. W. Churchman, *The Systems Approach,* New York, Dell Publishing, 1968. C. W. Churchman, *The Design of Inquiring Systems,* New York, Basic Books, Inc., 1971. S. Toulmin, *Human Understanding,* Oxford, Clarendon Press, 1972, Vol. 1.

24. E. Riska, "Paradigms in the Study of Health Policy," *Policy Studies Journal,* 1980-81, 9:2, Special No. 1, 198-212.

25. V. Navarro, *Medicine Under Capitalism,* New York, Prodist, 1976. V. Navarro, *Class Struggle, the State and Medicine: An Historical and Contemporary Analysis of the Medical Sector in Great Britain,* New York, Prodist, 1978.

26. A. C. Enthoven, "Consumer Choice Health Plan," *The New England Journal of Medicine,* March 23 and March 30, 1978, 650-658 and 709-720.

27. M. S. Feldstein, *Hospital Costs and Health Insurance,* Cambridge, Harvard University Press, 1981.

28. W. J. McNerny, "Control of Health Care Costs in the 1980's," *The New England Journal of Medicine,* Nov. 6, 1980, 1303:19, 1088-1095.

29. H. S. Luft, *Health Maintenance Organizations,* New York, John Wiley and Sons Inc., 1981.

30. L. F. Berkman and S. L. Syme, "Social Networks, Host Resistance and Mortality," *American Journal of Epidemiology,* 109:2, February 1979, 186-204.

31. J. W. Farquhar, et al., "Community Education for Cardiovascular Health," *Lancet,* 1:8023, June 4, 1977, 1192-95.

32. J. E. Fielding, "Success of Prevention," *Milbank Memorial Fund Quarterly,* 56, 1978, 432-435.

33. H. L. Blum, ibid, No. 3, 165-190.

INDEX

Index of Authors

Index of Content

STAPLE EDGE WHEN FOLDED

DETACH FROM BOOK, STAPLE EDGE WHEN FOLDED

MAKE YOUR OWN
POSTAGE-PREPAID ENVELOPE

DETACH THIS PAGE FROM THE BOOK, FILL OUT THE EVALUATION FORM ON BACK SIDE, FOLD SO THAT THE FORM IS INSIDE. STAPLE THE EDGES, AND MAIL. THANK YOU FOR YOUR HELP.

STAPLE EDGE WHEN FOLDED

DETACH FROM BOOK AND FOLD HERE, TO MAKE POSTAGE-FREE ENVELOPE

NO POSTAGE
NECESSARY
IF MAILED
IN THE
UNITED STATES

BUSINESS REPLY MAIL
FIRST CLASS PERMIT NO. **7670** OAKLAND, CA

Postage will be paid by addressee

THIRD PARTY PUBLISHING COMPANY
P.O. BOX 13306
MONTCLAIR STATION E
OAKLAND, CALIFORNIA 94661

EVALUATION: BLUM—EXPANDING HEALTH CARE HORIZONS, SECOND EDITION

EVALUATION FORM

We value your feedback. Please take a few moments to reflect on Dr. Henrik Blum's second edition of **Expanding Health Care Horizons** and give us your evaluation of it. Simply detach this form from the book, fold and seal it, and mail it to us. We pay the postage.

Date ____________________

	Check One				
	Very Poor	Poor	Fair	Good	Excellent
1. The book, in general	☐	☐	☐	☐	☐
2. Chapter 1. From our Understanding of Health, Health Care, and Medical Care to a National Health Policy	☐	☐	☐	☐	☐
3. Chapter 2. The Ecology of Health	☐	☐	☐	☐	☐
4. Chapter 3. Evidence Supporting a General Systems or Ecologic View of Health	☐	☐	☐	☐	☐
5. Chapter 4. Effective Health Care: The Required Processes and Relationships	☐	☐	☐	☐	☐
6. Chapter 5. One Example of a Delivery System that Meets our Requirements for Effective Health Care	☐	☐	☐	☐	☐
7. Chapter 6. Attributes and Training of the Professionals Working in the Primary Care Setting	☐	☐	☐	☐	☐
8. Chapter 7. A National Health Policy That Moves Us Towards Our Goals	☐	☐	☐	☐	☐
9. Chapter 8. Planning as a Tool of Social Change	☐	☐	☐	☐	☐

Comments: ____

____

____

May we quote you? ☐ Yes, ☐ No.

Use of the book (check the most appropriate response)

1) _____ I use it in my professional practice in the following manner: ____________________

____

____

2) _____ I use it in my teaching. Name of course: ____________________

____

No. of students ____________________

3) _____ I am a student, and am using it to: ____________________

____

____

Name: ____________________ Degree: __________

Title: ____

Address: ____

____

City ____________________ State __________ Zip __________

Thank you

Paul R. Mico, Publisher